Contents

Introduction 13

Brief History 15

ROOT CHAKRA - MULADHARA 19

SACRAL CHAKRA -SVADHISHTHANA 33

SOLAR PLEXUS CHAKRA - MANIPURA 48

HEART CHAKRA - ANAHATA 58

THROAT CHAKRA VISHUDDHA 73

THIRD EYE CHAKRA AJNA 85

CROWN CHAKRA SAHASRARA 97

Chakra Meditations 110

The Science Behind Chakra 111

How to maintain harmony and balance in your chakra......
121

Spirituality and connection to nature...................................
127

KUNDALINI..
132

Description...
133

Aura ....
150

CONCLUSION ....
157

Chakra for beginners

The ultimate guide to balancing, healing and unblocking your chakras, while gaining health and positive energy.

Healeanor Crystal

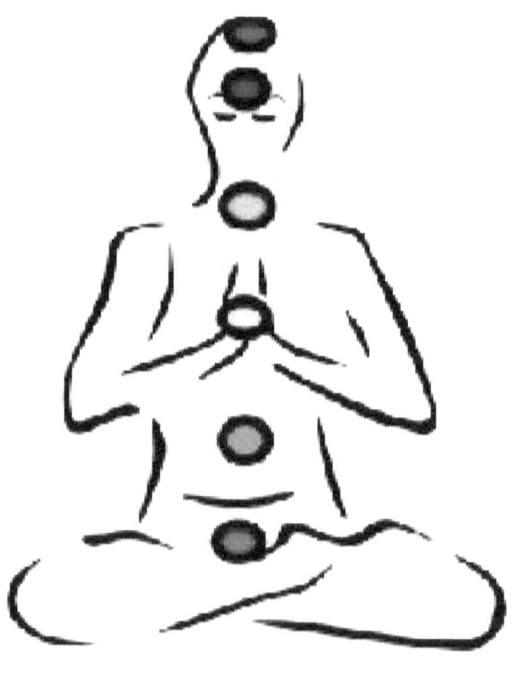

Illustration of seven main chakra points on human body

Introduction

What Are Chakras? The word chakra is derived from the Sanskrit word cakra, meaning "wheel." It was first mentioned in the Vedas, ancient Hindu texts that date to around 1,500 BCE. Chakras regulate your body energy levels, and how energy moves throughout.

You are already familiar with your physical body. You know how it feels to flex or extend an area of your body; that your muscles are attached to your bones; that your nerves signal to your limbs, torso, and head; and that what you eat and drink affects your health. In these ways, you can already see how aspects of your physical being are connected to each other, and how your perceptions through touch, smell, taste, sight, and hearing inform each other, creating your life experiences. However, your physical body is not the only body you have. Whether you're studying chakras or quantum physics, you come to learn that everything is energy, with its own vibrational frequency. From the most basic atoms that create our cells, organs, bones, muscles, and bodily systems to the most expansive planet in the solar system, everything is made up of energy. And that energy has many names: qi, ki, chi, prana, mana, Odic force, bioplasm, and life force energy, among many others. The energy body is the human energy field that extends beyond the physical body. Much as your physical body consists of many layers— your nervous system, musculature, and skeletal system— with intricate, overlapping functions, your energy body also consists of many interacting layers. Like your physical body, each layer serves a specific purpose and the layers work collectively as one. Together, the layers of your energy body are called your aura. Your aura interacts with your physical body as well as your energy centers, or chakras.

Chapter 1
Brief History

Throughout history, many cultures—including the Egyptians, Hindus, Chinese, Sufis, Zarathustrians, Greeks, Native Americans, Incas, and the Maya, among others—have all known these energy centers, or the chakra system, to be a reflection of the natural law that exists within the universe and an intertwined counterpart to our physical selves.

Chakras are energy vortexes that exist within each of us. These energy vortexes transport energy from the universe around you into your aura and body, as well as between the physical body and the layers of your aura. You can think of your chakra system as similar to a spiritual bloodstream. Blood carries oxygen, nutrients, and hormones throughout the body; helps regulate and balance the body; and protects the body by removing waste products and clotting when the body is harmed. Much in the same way your bloodstream connects and supports your many other physical bodily systems, your chakra system connects and supports your physical self and your energy self. All living things—humans, animals, plants, trees, even the Earth— have a chakra system, a living system of energy vortexes, that exists within them. The chakra system originated in India between 1500 and 500 BC in the oldest text called the Vedas.

Evidence of chakras, spelled cakra, is also found in the Shri Jabala Darshana Upanishad, the Cudamini Upanishad, the Yoga-Shikka Upanishad and the Shandilya Upanishad. According to the scholar Anodea Judith in her book the Wheels of Life, knowledge of the chakra system was passed down through an oral tradition by the Indo-Eurpoean people, also called the Aryan people. It was traditionally an Eastern philosophy until New Age authors, like Anodea Judith, resonated with the idea and wrote about the chakras.

There are seven major chakras in the body, as well as several minor ones. Each one is associated with specific organs and glands, physical functions and dysfunctions, and emotional, mental, and spiritual issues. We'll get into more specifics about each later in this chapter. When we get in touch with the energy within our chakras, we connect with ourselves more fully, and learn how to heal ourselves on all levels, creating true holistic healing. This is why mindfulness-based practices, such as meditation, help connect the mind with body and spirit, why certain physical activities can help clear your head and feel more centered, and why cultivating your spirit heals your mind and body. It is all connected.

Seven Main Chakras

1) Your Root chakra is an energy center located at your tailbone. The root chakra represents your connection to the Earth, your tribe or family, and survival issues.

2) The Sacral chakra is between your hips, a couple inches below your navel. The Sacral chakra represents creativity, manifestation, sexuality, and emotional connection to others.

3) The Solar chakra is located in the center of your torso, about six inches below your heart.

4) Your Heart chakra is located in the center of your chest. The heart chakra represents unconditional love, nurturing, and compassion.

5) Next is the Throat chakra. The throat chakra represents communication, expression of feelings, your ability to effectively convey the meaning of your words.

6) The Third eye is located low on the forehead, a little above your eyebrows. The Third eye represents insight, intuition, wisdom, intelligence, and psychic development

7) The last primary energy center, the Crown chakra, is located a couple inches above the top of your head. The Crown chakra represents spirituality and connectedness to all things.

If a chakra is out of balance, your health in that area will be out balance. For instance, if your heart chakra is overactive, you will try to fall in love without healthy boundaries. If your heart chakra is underactive, you will be unable to love yourself or feel love for others. I think of it as an energetic way of looking at overall health and well-being. It's incredibly consistent, in my opinion. An understanding of the chakra system makes it much easier to deduce where your imbalances may be. If you have heart disease, you probably have an imbalance in your heart chakra. If you have poor eyesight, it's likely an imbalance in your third eye. As a nutritionist and an energy worker, I have oftentimes been able to help people heal themselves through awareness of the 7 chakra system.

As with all bodily systems; cardiovascular system, immune system, etc., all of these 7 chakras interact with one another, like wheels. The balance of one affects the balance of the others. They're all connected, a part of the whole.

Chapther 2

ROOT CHAKRA - MULADHARA

This chakra is the first of the seven major chakras (or energy vortices) which play such a key role in the energetic functioning of the body. It is situated at the base of the spine in the perineal area, and is also known as the root chakra, or by its Sanskrit name 'Muladhara'.

The root chakra is all about being grounded, feeling secure that your basic needs are being met, and feeling connected to your family and tribal consciousness in healthy ways. This first chakra is strongly linked with physical survival, and maintaining a sense of stability and security.

It is associated with the colour red, and is symbolised by a four-petalled lotus flower. In a balanced state, this chakra promotes a sense of groundedness, as well as a strong sense of individuality. It is also linked with security-related issues such as financial prosperity.

If its healthy balance is disturbed, this may manifest as feelings of insecurity or even fear, a dulled survival instinct, as well as anger and physical problems such as back pain, knee trouble and issues with the lower digestive system.

Identifying Blocked Root Charka and symptoms

You can tell if your root chakra is closed if

- You feel you have to survive life and are constantly getting by or going without

- You often feel stuck and sluggish

- You experience unrelenting stress because of a belief that you must rely on external circumstances

- You feel you have been abandoned by your parents

- You may have persistant financial problems and find yourself in a less-than-ideal career

- You hate your body and feel you are not good enough the way you are.

You don't think you have enough money:
While a blocked root chakra is very common for those suffering from extreme financial crisis, most people who are extremely rich also suffer from this problem. That's why they evade taxes, squirrel away their money behind shell companies, and stress out over not having enough villas and Ferraris.

You are a shopaholic:
Whether you like cars or perfumes, if you own one too many things and can't stop yourself from buying more, it's a clear sign you are trying to plug your insecurities with superficial possessions.

You have anger issues:
If you have a habit of lashing out at people, stonewalling them, or holding onto bitter grudges, it's because you felt the situation shouldn't have happened the way it did and the person who wronged you shouldn't have behaved in such a manner.
And frankly, that's laughable. Why? Because we have zero control over people and life. Nevertheless, if you persist in trying to control people and your surroundings, it's a big sign that you are unstable and insecure on the inside.

Physical Symptoms Include:
Lethargy, cold hands and feet, Lower back pain, Constipation, Knee issues, Bone issues, Kidney stones, Feet issues, Urinary issues, Colon issues, Leg issues, any issues from the base of your spine and down.

Emotional Symptoms Include:
Eating disorders, Inability to focus or sit still, Lacking energy, Feeling ungrounded and floating high, Craving comfort foods, Fear of job instability, Desire to be outside more, Drawn to the color red,

Not feeling secure in life, Co-dependency, Lack of focus.

The root chakra is located at the base of your spine, or tailbone. The root chakra belongs to the realm of the physical. If you feel grounded, secure, and rooted in the present, this chakra needs little attention. However, many are not so blessed. A blocked root chakra may lead you to grasp at the physical, becoming clingy and overly possessive. An imbalance in the root chakra can also lead to anxiety disorders, fears and nightmares. Conversely, if you're too open here you may feel estranged from your body and possessions. As a result, your generosity may be taken advantage of.

Balancing your root chakra

1. Get on your yoga mat. Many yoga postures are designed to cleanse this chakra. My favorite is tree pose. You can use your 'seeing red' visualization as you firmly plant your entire left foot onto your mat and bring your right foot up into tree pose. Keep your hip points squarely ahead and your toes tucked in as you place your foot anywhere on your leg besides your knee. Be creative and make your tree pose your own. Place your right leg into half lotus or engage your core and reach your arms overhead, keeping the base of your neck soft and your elbows straight as you rotate the pinky side of your hands in to engage your triceps. Most importantly, feel supported and connected to the earth as you hold your tree pose for 5 to 8 breaths before switching sides.

2. See red. Seriously—envisioning the color red glowing brightly at the base of the spine, where this chakra is located, is the beginning of root chakra cleansing and balancing. Start with the simple meditation of imaging a bright red light at

the base of your tailbone. Picture this red light extending down your legs and feet, grounding you to the earth.

3. Take a shower. This is such a wonderful root chakra cleanser. We are physical animals in addition to being intelligent, thoughtful human beings. Embrace and love your physicality by being completely present as you bathe. Mindfully moving is a powerful form of meditation.

4. Get a pedicure. I had to throw this one in. My grandfather had a friend that was known for saying, "you can always tell how well a person takes care of themselves by how they take care of their feet." This might be a little bit of an exaggeration, but loving your feet and taking the time to pamper your physical body are great ways to also care for your root chakra energy.

5. Zen out on a walk. Take this idea of mindfully moving on your walk with you. Concentrate on your foot leaving the ground and connecting to the earth again with each step. You'll give your mind a break and cleanse your root chakra at the same time.

6. Toning: Using the sound LAM, or use Do from the "Do, Re, Mi" scale

The Root Chakra is the foundation of your energetic 'house'. It draws energy from the Earth to nourish and energize your body. When the Root is compromised, the energy flow to the other chakras may be impacted as well. It is therefore essential to build a strong foundation to overall stability and health.

Healing your root chakra

Basically, each chakra has a diverse benefits for your bodily and emotional well-being. Preferably, you'll develop techniques for all of the chakras at some point, but it's wise to start with the foundational one. Learning how to open the root chakra, in particular, is fairly straightforward, but it can have profound impacts on how you feel. You can improve your self-confidence, feel more ready to face your feels, experience a deeper sense of relaxation, and feel more engaged in fun or playful interactions. The basic sense of stability that you cultivate will permeate all aspects of your life.

These are some techniques for unblocking the root chakra, offering concrete advice for integrating each exercise into your daily life.

Root Chakra Meditation And Yoga Techniques:
When it comes to overall healing, root chakra meditations can also help you. Chakra meditation techniques are very much like regular meditation techniques, but with a focus on one specific area of the body.

Sit with your shoulders back and your spine straight. Try to relax all your muscles as you close your eyes and breathe deeply. Inhale through the nose, pulling the breath as far down into your body as you can, and exhale through the mouth.

Turn your attention to the location of the root chakra, right below your tailbone. Notice any tightness in the area.

Since the root chakra's element is red, try picturing a red glow at the base of your spine. This glow will slowly expand, making the whole area warm and relaxed. Rest in this sensation for 3-5 minutes.

When you're ready, slowly open your eyes. Sit for a few minutes before continuing with your day.

Some yoga poses are also linked to your root chakra's functionality. For example, root chakra yoga poses include Balasana, which involves lying face down, resting on your knees and calves, then extending your arms out in front of you as your head drops down between them.

Chakra Foods List And Diet Suggestions:

Other chakra exercises involve making small changes to your diet. Experts on rebalancing and opening the chakras are increasingly interested in the impact food can have on your alignment and vibration. Firstly, you'll typically find that a healthy diet helps to keep your chakras open. This means reducing levels of salt, sugar and saturated fats, and increasing your intake of fruits and vegetables.

However, there are also specific foods that are linked to the root chakra. Anything organic is an excellent option because the root chakra is opened by anything connected to our tribal roots. In addition:

Protein-rich foods help to ground you and give you physical strength, which then helps to boost emotional strength. Good examples include beans, tofu, green peas, spinach, and almonds.

Red foods automatically influence your root chakra because of its association with the color red. These foods usually give you lots of vitamin C, as a bonus. Think of strawberries, cherries, tomatoes and red bell peppers.

Root vegetables like beets, garlic, and potatoes are all grounding too, partly because they grow in the soil. This link to the earth foundations means they can also help to rebalance a misaligned chakra.

Root Chakra Affirmations To Use:

Finally, targeted affirmations are incredibly useful for root chakra healing. As with all affirmations, you can repeat these positive statements multiple times a day, or anytime you get a sense your chakra might be blocked. In particular, you might want to try saying one or more of these root chakra affirmations right before or after you meditate, or when you get ready for the day ahead.

- "Wherever I am, I am safe and secure."

- "I am stable, grounded and relaxed in this moment."

- "All of my safety needs will always be met."

- "I have a healthy body, a healthy mind, and an abundant life."

- "I am anchored to the earth and supported by the universe."

- "The universe will always support me and show me where to go next."

- "I deserve and receive support whenever I need it."

- "The universe will always provide for me."

- "I feel my root chakra opening, and I feel myself stabilizing."

- "I am secure and happy in my home."

You can also combine affirmations with yoga poses, or try holding one of your root chakra stones while saying an affirmation. Some people also like to write their affirmations down, placing them in a prominent place as they continue daily chakra work.

Jewelry and stone for chakra

Influencing chakras often involves using unique stones, sometimes in the form of jewelry. By simply wearing or holding these stones, you may be able to realign or begin to unblock a troubled chakra. However, each chakra is associated with different stone. Colors and gems can help bring a chakra into balance. The root chakra's color is red. Gemstones for the first chakra include garnet, red jasper, black tourmaline, obsidian, and bloodstone. You can place the gemstone on the area of the chakra while lying down to help open and align it.

Red Jasper. The root chakra's associated color is red, so it's no surprise that many of the root chakra stones are red as we. This one is linked to balancing, so it's an ideal stone to have if you are battling erratic mood swings.

Red Carnelian. A pale red stone with orange hues, red carnelian is associated with strength, cleansing, and bravery. It is a good choice if you particularly struggle with fearfulness and can't bring yourself to leave your comfort zone.

Obsidian. A black gemstone, obsidian is said to protect you from harm. You may draw some comfort from wearing it as you work to move to a place of greater security in your life.

Bloodstone. The stone itself is green. The name refers to its red spots. This semi-precious stone is linked to pushing away negative energy and increasing confidence. A perfect stone for combatting significant root chakra blocks.

Black Tourmaline — Black — Semi-precious — Used for spiritual grounding, this stone is good for cleansing and balancing.

For thousands of years, light workers and energy healers have used specific stones to calm and focus the mind, reduce stress, and foster health and vitality.

Lifestyle and diet consideration

- Eat root vegetables, which will help ground you.

- Take some time to do activities where your bare feet are planted into the earth, soil, or sand.

- Spend some time in nature.

- Make pottery (this will help your sacral plexus chakra, too).

- Stomp your feet to connect with the earth or ground (even if you're in a building).

Mantra for root chakra

Chanting or toning sounds can also help bring you back to balance just like music brings people together. Sounds create vibrations in the body, and these vibrations help the cells work together in synchronistic harmony. The mantra sound that corresponds to the root chakra is LAM.

Chapter 3

SACRAL CHAKRA - SVADHISHTHANA

This Chakra is the second chakra and is located below the belly button in the lower abdomen, and its color is orange.

The color orange is associated with vitality, endurance, creativity, enthusiasm and joy. It symbolizes energy, warmth, and the sun. But orange is a little less intensity or aggression than red as it is softened by the inclusion of yellow.

Organs associated with this are the uterus, ovaries, testes, large bowel, prostate and circulation. If you suffer from pre-menstrual tension, ovarian cysts, irritable bowel syndrome, endometriosis, low back pain, pancreatic or testicular diseases then this is the chakra you need to work on.

It also represents the aspect of self acceptance, allowing ourselves to be who we really are, self-respect and from this flows respect for others. Self-acceptance is accepting and loving ourselves as we are now. We may have things we want to change but while they are part of us we need to learn to love and accept them. It is only as we learn to totally accept ourselves that we are then able to accept others.

This is our relationship center and determines how well we are able to equally give and receive. It is the center of our passion for life.

This center is also responsible for duality. When opposites within us and our emotions balance each other, the relationship is healthy, and we are but, when there are extremes of either polarity then problems can occur. In it's extreme this is Bipolar disorder. It is also when this center is unbalanced that our thoughts and feelings can lead to depression, additions and anorexia or bulimia.

The Sanskrit name for this one is Svadisthana, which translates as "sacred home of the self." I love this as we so often forget that we are sacred and we need to honor ourselves and this is the center where we do this. In females this rotates clockwise and for men, anticlockwise. This energy center is about going with the flow, accepting things as they are, just being and being in the moment.

The color of this chakra speaks to me of sunrise and sunset. Most people when they stop to observe these, let go of everything and are just 'in the moment'. It also speaks of hope, hope for what the new day will bring or the hope of tomorrow. This energy vortex is where our poetic skills come from.

Identifying blocked Sacral chakra and symptoms

- You experience difficulty allowing yourself to become emotionally and sexually intimate

- You believe sex is bad and that it can hurt you, or your feel you have to be sexy to be loved

- You feel abused, hurt, and confused and don't trust that you can be loved for being you

- You struggle with a healthy self-image

- You move from one relationship to another, desperately trying to find "the one" yet lacking the sense that you are worthy of love.

- feeling unemotional

- feeling guarded

- not feeling excited about anything

- feeling unable to focus

- feeling out of touch with creative side

- experiencing self-deprivation

- feeling detached

- feeling insecure

- experiencing low self-esteem

- experiencing sexual repression

- feeling jealous often

- comparing yourself to others

- displaying poor social skills

- feeling fearful

- feeling aloof often

- feeling shy or timid

- denying yourself of pleasure

- feeling overwhelmingly exhausted

- feeling a lack of desire

- feeling a lack of passion.

Balancing your sacral chakra

A blockage of energy in the sacral chakra can be healed with regular practice designed to stimulate the chakra, which allows energy to flow into it and excess energy to dissipate. Chakra balancing can be helped along by a healer, but there are many things you can do on your own as well.

Aromatherapy:

Sandalwood, Ylang-ylang, Neroli, Orange, Tangerine, Geranium, Rose, Rosemary, Jasmine.
These essential oils can be used in several ways. My favorite is the easiest—use a diffuser. This can be as easy as a drop of essential oil on a cotton ball that is placed where you can sniff it. I have a diffuser that goes on for five minutes every twenty-five minutes. I use this one at night. If you work in an office, they now make diffusers with a USB you can plug into your computer. The scents stay close and are relatively unobtrusive to those working around you.
Body oils and lotions are easy as well, just ensure that only pure essential oils and not chemical fragrance oils are the main ingredients.
An aromatherapy bath with bath salts can be made with any of the oils above, or a blend. (If you're new to blending, start with two or three oils or you might be unhappy with the result). The bath should be exotic - neroli is preferable, but you can add a drop

of mandarin orange or sandalwood, clary sage, patchouli, or cinnamon. Use orange candles (scented with essential oils) and use soft music with water sounds.

You can also diffuse a drop of your oil of choice on a pad and inserted into an aromatherapy necklace

Since the element of this chakra is water, music with sounds of the ocean, a waterfall or rainfall in the background might be a good choice for you.

Nature Therapy:

Water is the element associated with the sacral chakra. Being close to the ocean, a lake, or even the rain are all immensely beneficial. Allow the flow of water to mirror the way your life. If you don't have any nearby, a fountain will work nearly as well. and your life-giving energy flows through you with ease, joy, purpose, and pleasure. Even taking a simple bath or a shower can help calm and release the energy flow.

Wearing orange to help feel open and creative, or if you look awful in orange, wear orange jewelry under your blouse.

Exercise:

Another way to help your sacral back into balance is to dance! Five minutes of your favorite dance every day will certainly help maintain balance! Longer is better, of course!

Yoga poses can also help. Try out the triangle, pigeon pose, kneeling crescent moon, fish pose, and bridge poses.

Nutrition Therapy:
As always, a well-balanced diet is the most important thing. If you can, work with a nutritionist and your health care professional to determine if you are lacking in some nutrient and what you need in order to improve the condition.

Since this is the water element, be sure to drink lots of liquids—juices (with minimal sugar), tea, coffee (in moderation), and water. Consume fresh fruits that are juicy, e.g., oranges, papayas, mangos, melons, strawberries, tangerines, apricots, passion fruit, and cranberries. Smoothies with tropical fruits are a summer treat.

Eat a lot of vegetables, especially orange ones, e.g., yams, sweet potatoes, squash, pumpkin and carrots are especially helpful.

Healing your sacral chakra

Healing Foods:

Orange colored foods like oranges and tangerines.

Meditation for healing the Sacral chakra:

Meditation is very useful for chakra cleansing and balancing. For example, a simple sacral chakra healing meditation consists in envisioning an orange lotus or orange crescent moon in the area of the second chakra in the pelvis area. Hold that image in your mind for a few minutes while breathing deeply.

Imagine a warm glowing ball of orange light in the middle of a beautiful glowing lotus right below your naval. Imagine the lotus blooming and shedding its beautiful light across your lower back, sex organs, and abdomen. Next, image the orange flower blooming into a bright orange crescent moon. Hold that image in your sacral and take five deep breaths. Feel the energy flow through you and warm you with safety, warmth, creativity, and pleasure.

Yoga for healing the Sacral chakra:

The hips are heavily affected by the sacral chakra. When using yoga to heal the sacral, focus on opening the hips with triangle pose and bound angle pose. Practice in a calm place where you can go slowly and at your own pace.

Kneel and slide a block between your heels, so that the short edges of the block center on your ankles; sit back and press the tops of your feet and toenails evenly into the ground. Now sit tall, lengthening the crown of your head upward. Make sure the block evenly supports both sitting bones. Place your hands on your thighs or over your belly as you roll your shoulder heads back, then make your belly round with each full inhale. After a few breaths, start to cultivate Ujjayi Pranayama (Victorious Breath) by sweeping your breath along the back of your throat as you inhale and exhale through the nose. Stay here for 2 to 3 minutes. By beginning in this posture, you set a grounding tone for your practice. From Virasana, walk your hands forward into Tabletop, with your knees under your hips, and your wrists under your shoulders. Make small circles with your hips, warming up the spine and inviting a sense of fluidity. As you grow warmer, you can expand your circles, to the point of melting all the way back into Balasana (Child's Pose) for a few breaths. Spend at least 1 minute circling in each direction. When you are done, lift your hips back into Adho Mukha Svanasana (Downward-Facing Dog Pose).

Anjaneyasana:
From Down Dog, step your right foot toward your right thumb tip and set your back knee on the mat. Press the top of your foot firmly into the mat as you lengthen your tailbone toward your mat and draw your low belly in. Make sure your front knee doesn't drift past your front ankle. Extend your arms alongside your ears. Interlace all but your index fingers, and press up through your palms, drawing

your shoulders away from your ears. Bring your drishti, or gaze, up as you lift from your sternum and breathe underneath your collarbones. Firmly draw your hips in toward your midline as you grow tall through the sides of your waist and up through your index fingers. Hold for 1 minute.

Ardha Hanumanasana:
From Low Lunge, lower your hands to either side of your right foot and shift back, straightening your right leg and flexing your right foot. Lengthen your heart forward on the inhale and fold on the exhale; if you feel your lower back rounding during this action, slide blocks underneath your palms or tent your fingertips. Move with the breath, playing with a wavelike movement of the upper body for 10 to 12 breaths. Then exhale to press back to Down Dog, and take Low Lunge and Half Splits on the left side. Finish in Down Dog.

Utkata Konasana: From Down Dog, come to standing and bring your feet one leg's distance apart; spin your legs and toes out about 45 degrees. Bend your knees deeply to create a 90-degree angle between your *q*uads and shins, and press your knees open so that they align directly with the center of your feet. Draw your low belly in and your tailbone down. Position your torso right over your pelvis as you reach the crown of your head toward the sky. Place your palms together at your heart in Anjali Mudra (Salutation Seal). Try to hold this posture for 1 minute; while you breathe here, find organic movement as you shift slightly from side to side, or even forward and back, grounding through your heels and toes.

Virabhadrasana II: From Goddess, turn your hips to the right as you spin your back heel and plant it flat on the mat, parallel to the short edge of your mat or with left toes turned in just slightly. Line up your front heel with the arch of your back foot. Extend evenly through both arms and hands. Direct your gaze over your right middle finger. Move your right knee directly over your right ankle, aligning your knee in the direction of your second and third toes. Breathe for 6 to 8 full cycles. As you lunge forward in this powerful standing posture, remain receptive to all that's occurring within you. Allow sensations, thoughts, and emotions to move through you with ease by simply reminding yourself that each experience is impermanent.

Affirmations:
- I welcome healthy change.
- I am flexible.
- I embrace my sexuality.
- My emotions are healthy.

Jewelry and stone for sacral chakra

The chakra color for Swadhisthana is orange and it is tied to the moon, so orange and yellow gems are good for opening the sacral chakra. Gems in opposite colors can be used to soothe an overactive sacral chakra.

Crystals that open and activate the second chakra include:

- Orange and coral calcite
- Citrine
- Orange carnelian
- Orange adventurine

Orange calcite and citrine both have cleansing properties, which can help clear a blockage in the chakra. Coral calcite is often used in distance healing because of its amplifying qualities.

If your second chakra is overactive, stones that can be used to soothe it include:

- Orange carnelian
- Snowflake obsidian
- Amber
- Purple gemstones like amethyst, **q**uartz and tourmaline

Orange carnelian can be used for either opening or soothing because of its unique healing properties. Amber chakra stones are known for drawing energy into themselves, so can be used to soak up excess energy in the

second chakra. Snowflake obsidian restores balance to the body.

Moonstone is a unique crystal because it can be used for both opening and soothing the sacral chakra because of its connection with the moon, which is also associated with the second chakra. The meaning of moonstone varies slightly depending on the variety, but all are good for the sacral chakra, especially ones with a slight golden or yellow hue.

Lifestyle and diet consideration

- Dance—especially belly dancing, Latin dances such as salsa, and other dances that move the hip area.

- Practice hula-hooping.

- Learn tantra to get in touch with your sexuality on a more conscious level.

- Try journaling, writing, painting, or another form of creative expression to help channel your emotions.

- Learn how to express your emotions in healthy ways.

- Include play in your daily life to cultivate flexibility in learning how to experience pleasure and joy.

Take the following food

- Oranges

- Mangos

- Carrots

- Pumpkin

- Dark Chocolate

- Sweet Potatoes (try them mashed with butter and cinnamon)

- Cantaloupe

- Peaches

- Figs (fresh, not dried)

Mantra for Sacral chakra

VAM is the Chakra Mantra for the Sacral. It's actually pronounced Vang!

Chapter 4

SOLAR PLEXUS CHAKRA - MANIPURA

The solar plexus chakra is all about standing in your power, getting in touch with your inner warrior fire, and self-esteem.

Identifying blocked Solar plexus chakra ans symptoms

Symptoms of blockage:
It's easy for the solar plexus to become blocked because of the many overwhelming options life throws at you.
When you don't know what you want, when you're fearful of making wrong decisions, when you need input and buy-in from others to move forward, this chakra gets blocked.
Emotional signs of a Blockage:
 Sometimes the symptoms of chakra blockage can be subtle, but not so much with the solar plexus chakra. It's often easy to see and tune into once you're aware. If you lack confidence, if you struggle to

make things happen for yourself, if you feel like you're always being pushed around by others, if you're waiting for someone to offer you a leadership role, or if you're exhausted from always trying too hard, it's likely that your solar plexus is blocked.

You can also see when your personal power chakra is blocked if you generally feel unworthy, you constantly second guess yourself, you carry a strong sense of victimhood, and you feel powerless against the wants and needs of the people in your life.

Physical Indications of a Blocked Solar Plexus Chakra:

An excess of energy in the solar plexus leads to overeating and general overindulgence in things. Laziness, a need to control, intolerance, and competition are more signs of an excess of energy in the solar plexus chakra.

An energetic deficiency in the solar plexus manifests as low body weight, lack of focus, and digestive problems like ulcers or indigestion.

Deficiencies in the solar plexus often mean that you struggle to represent yourself honestly. You may have difficulties knowing yourself and what you really want.

With a blocked or out of balanced solar plexus chakra, you're not able to define your will or direction and therefore procrastinate on major life decisions.

Balancing Solar plexus chakra

There are as many different ways to balance our chakras as there are people in the world, and what works for one person may not work for another. Some people like to sit and meditate, using sounds and smells to relax and re-energize, while others may chose exercise or participating in other activities that stimulate our points. Whichever way you chose, make sure that it's right for you. If you feel uncomfortable doing a yoga position, try listening to music and focusing on how your body responds, or if you are more energetic, a good hike or riding a bike might be better suited. This is the important part; listen to your body. It will tell you what works and what doesn't.

To nourish your spiritual side, try volunteering or taking a class; learn something new. This nourishes our mind and spirit.

Crystals:
Stones of yellow hue are best to use. Crystals such as amber, citrine, golden or honey calcite, yellow sapphire are just a few. Wear or place these crystals on your body as you listen to meditative music, or carry them in your pocket.

Sound:
Using sound as part of your chakra balancing is a soothing and relaxing way to release the tension and

blockage within our bodies. Either by 'toning' which is using a specific vowel sound, drawing it out in a tone of voice you feel comfortable using. For the Solar Plexus, the sound of 'oh' should be used. A Bijas mantra is different and can be used as well. The Bijas for the Solar Plexus is RAM.

New Experiences:
The Solar Plexus helps with mental clarity as well as learning new things. Try taking up a new hobby or playing games that stimulate and sharpens your mind. These are excellent ways to keep this chakra open and balanced.

While the majority of these suggestions concentrate with feeding our emotional and mental side, we need to think of our body as well. Keeping the body healthy with the right food and good exercise can also keep the chakras balanced and the energy flowing. Consider eating foods that are yellow, such as some squash, yellow bell peppers and lemons. Fruits and vegetables of this color contain antioxidants such as lutein. Research suggests that lutein along with other plant basted antioxidants, may reduce the risk of chronic eye disease.

Healing your Solar plexus chakra

It's a good idea to devote time to learning techniques focused on each of the 7 chakras. Each one offers its own benefits. That said, there are clear advantages to focusing merely on the solar plexus chakra, at least for a time. When you work on creating a more positive self-image, on making responsible decisions and on understanding what you want from life, good things follow!

Whether you want to find a relationship, get more job satisfaction or broaden your social life, confidence and autonomy are necessary precursors. You will also likely experience psychological or spiritual growth, and, as a bonus, notice smoother digestion and less stomach discomfort.

Since the solar plexus chakra also has a lot to do with life purpose, working on this chakra can also reduce procrastination. Similarly, it can help you ensure you're using your time to create a better future for yourself. We'll turn now to look at four specific ways in which you can unblock your solar plexus chakra. Remember to consider how you can integrate these techniques into your everyday life.

As you probably know, all stones and crystals have ancient meanings and associations. As such, it's unsurprising that there are stones allocated to each chakra.

You can use these stones in a variety of ways when

opening chakras. You might wear solar plexus chakra jewelry, hold a stone in the palm of your hand when meditating, or simply carry one in your pocket to help keep your solar plexus in alignment.

Yoga for solar plexus:

You can also add yoga poses to your day if you want to align or unblocked the solar plexus chakra. Experts on chakra work typically encourage all forms of yoga, but particular exercises are more influential on the position of the solar plexus chakra. For example, try the child's pose, which also offers the advantage of being very soothing:

• Put a soft blanket or cushion under your knees.

• Kneel down, sitting on your heels

• Move your knees so they are hip-width apart.

• Lean down so your torso sits between your thighs.

Jewelry and stone for Solar plexus chakra

Here are the stones most frequently associated with solar plexus chakra:

Amber:

Your solar plexus chakra is marked as yellow on maps of the chakras, so yellow is often used to symbolize it more generally. Amber stones are an orangey-yellow in color, and they are linked to both confidence and mental clarity. Use this stone if you're struggling to make a decision.

Yellow tourmaline:

Yellow tourmaline is physically striking, and you'll often see it advertised as a "detox" stone on a list of solar plexus crystals. It's all about getting rid of negativity (both in views of yourself and the past).

Citrine:

Another yellow solar plexus crystal, this pale stone is sometimes called the "success stone". Any journey related to personal empowerment goes well with acquiring a piece of citrine, and you can also use citrine for self-esteem.

Lifestyle and diet consideration

Engage in the following activities:
- Wear yellow clothing.

- Take martial arts (internal or external), which helps strengthen personal power.

- Create healthy energy boundaries with those in your life to strengthen your inner power.

- A simple way to create an energy boundary is by surrounding yourself in an egg of white light, especially if you're about to enter a stressful situation, such as a talk with a toxic coworker, or, if you experience social anxiety, before entering a large room full of people.

- Try things outside your comfort zone. Doing so helps you build confidence in your own resilience.

Just as your diet influences your general health, so too does it impact on the seven major energy centers in your body. Consequently, one of the easiest ways to make a difference to chakra alignment is to tweak your diet so that it nurtures (rather than blocks) the chakras.

Increasing fiber intake, cutting back on sugar and reducing the amount of saturated fat in your diet are all great for your chakras. However, there are also particular chakra foods that target the solar plexus and can speed up solar plexus chakra healing:

Yellow peppers: Since yellow is the color of the solar plexus chakra, you can't go wrong when adding more yellow peppers to your diet.

Complex carbohydrates: Given that the solar plexus chakra plays a big role in the energy you have for pursuing goals, it's smart to go for food that gives you a steady, sustained supply of energy instead of just a spike in blood sugar. Good examples include brown rice, brown bread, and wholegrain cereal.

Corn: Another bright, optimistic yellow food, corn can nourish the solar plexus chakra and give your well-being an extra boost. It is often the first solar plexus food mentioned in a beginner's guide to chakras.

Chamomile tea: While not strictly a food, chamomile tea has always been recommended to help treat a solar plexus chakra blockage. It can also settle an unsettled stomach.

Mantra for Solar plexus chakra

The bij mantra that goes with this chakra is "rung" or "ram." Chanting this mantra can help awaken and ignite the solar plexus chakra. If you prefer English, you can also chant the affirmation, "I can" or "I do," either aloud or consciously silently.

As you chant the mantra, you can also try the hakini mudra. Bring the tips of all 5 fingers to touch, with the thumb and pinkie fingers nearly in line with each other. Hold the mudra in front of your solar plexus as you chant the bij mantra or meditate. Alternatively, try the rudra mudra, with your pointer and ring finger curled in to meet your thumb and your pinkie and middle finger extended.

Chapter 5

HEART CHAKRA - ANAHATA

Heart chakra is the middle chakra in a system of seven. It is related to love and is the integrator of opposites in the psyche: mind and body, male and female, persona and shadow, ego and unity. A healthy fourth chakra allows us to love deeply, feel compassion, and have a deep sense of peace and centeredness.

The 4th chakra: Anahata or Heart chakra is the balance point that involves the whole self. Your ability to feel love for yourself and for others. On a truly holistic level, the heart is your ability to see your connection to all that is. Ultimately, a perfectly balanced heart results in feeling genuine and unconditional love for all things. Your fourth chakra is located in the center of your chest, level with your heart.

a) Central powerhouse of the human energy system - the emotional power chakra - mediates between body and spirit and determines their health and strength. The symbolic doorway into our internal world.

b) Propels our emotional development - how to act out of love and compassion - to recognize that the most powerful energy we have is love.

c) To generate an emotional climate and steadiness with which we respond to experience/circumstance.

d) To let go and let God - to be able to see our experiences and circumstances as part of the divine plan.

e) Openness trust toward life - ego and will to outer world.

f) Getting to know ourselves in relationship to ourselves alone, not in regards to anyone else.

g) The ability to heal oneself and others.

h) Love recognized as commitment to self-love as primary factor for healthy relationships with others - love of self, forgiveness, compassion - a force that influences and determines biological activity - heals us and others.

Love is Divine power. Love is the only authentic power. Not only our minds and spirits, but also our physical bodies need love to survive and thrive. To refine our capacity to love others as well as ourselves and to develop the power of forgiveness (acceptance). The Heart Chakra governs the physical heart and lungs. It is essential to our physical supply of energy and vitality as well as the love that nourishes our spiritual existence. Centering ourselves in love gives our life purpose and meaning. It anchors us in Selfhood, which is love itself. What this means on a real level it is our true nature that is loving, kind, and respectful. Growth and healing open a panorama, where we give love freely and unconditionally and receive it in the same way.

Identifying blocked Heart chakra and symptoms

Symptoms of blockage:
Every chakra moves out of alignment at times or develops blockages. These blockages can be minor or major, but will always lead you to feel physically or emotionally off balance. Blocked heart chakra symptoms include the following:
- Restlessness
- Difficulty trusting others
- Impatience and irritability
- Lack of empathy

Some of the physical symptoms of a blocked heart chakra can include these (though note that these issues can, of course, have purely biological roots):
- Insomnia
- Increase in blood pressure
- A decrease in immune system function

There will be times when you don't know exactly what has gone wrong with your heart chakra. Healing doesn't require that you know the cause. That said, there are some common reasons why you might need to work on healing the heart chakra.

Difficult relationships are the main cause. These need not be romantic. Toxic friendships are just as capable of blocking the heart chakra.

You might be dealing with the end of a relationship, or with an imbalanced relationship where your love doesn't seem to be reciprocated. Any kind of grief or loss can also mean you need to practice heart chakra healing exercises.

In addition, if you're struggling to accept a truth about yourself, this type of emotional repression can also push the heart chakra out of alignment.

Balancing the Heart Chakra

Green Heals the Heart: Green is the color associated with the Fourth Chakra.

When you bring yourself to surroundings where green is plentiful – such as the trees and plants in nature – your Heart Chakra will feel at peace, allowing for healing to occur.

Green candles, green pictures or paintings, and even green painted walls can open up a closed Heart Chakra when outside nature cannot be explored.

Choose green foods on your plate – spinach, kale, swiss chard, romaine lettuce, parsley, bok choy, limes, green apples, honeydew melons, avocados, green peppers, cucumbers, and the like, all help balance the Heart Chakra.

Use the Element of Air:

Air is the element of the Heart Chakra, so surround yourself with this element often to help the Anahata thrive.

Walking on the beach or in the open plains, where the air can brush against your face – even feeling the breeze from an open window in your home – will do wonders for the Heart Chakra!

Practice meditation and the YAM chanting for a few minutes each day, along with verbal affirmations ("My heart is full. I am love. I forgive. I can heal.") for healing.

When we allow our hearts be open to love, forgiveness, and compassion, our Heart Chakra will become open as well.

Never forget what the Heart Chakra truly and naturally represents – LOVE.

Practice a random act of kindness every day, forgive easily, and love all who enter your life (for the good and the bad).

With these actions and intentions, your Heart Chakra will remain open, balanced, and alive.

Healing your Heart chakra

Here are the best heart chakra healing practices out there which will help you balance this energy center:

Go forest bathing:
As green is the color of the heart chakra, going out in nature will help your heart to open. "Forest bathing" is actually a term that originated in Japan known as Shinrin Yoku, and it has many scientifically proven benefits. If you don't live near a forest, don't worry. Simply go to your local park, woodland, bushland or other areas full of greenery. If you live in a city with no nature, try getting a pot plant or indoor shrubs to encourage heart chakra healing.

Do a loving-kindness meditation:
A balanced heart is beautiful. It dissolves the illusion of separateness and shares loving kindness with others. If your heart chakra feels congested, try the loving kindness meditation. Simply sit down in a *q*uiet spot and connect with your breath. Allow your chest area to soften as you direct loving energy towards yourself. Afterward, choose four different types of people to direct loving energy towards including a loved one, a person close to you, a neutral person (like an acquaintance), and an enemy or hostile person. You might like to visualize loving energy or say a mantra such as "I radiate love to you" to assist with this meditation.

Establish clear personal boundaries:
Examine where in your life you are permitting other people to overstep your boundaries. At what times do you say "yes" when you desperately want to say "no"? Which people in your life ask too much from you? In which areas of your life do you feel anxious and ungrounded? Develop the habit of drawing the line and respectfully letting people know where your limits are. Practice assertiveness and take care of yourself.

Use the following herbs:
Use herbs such as rose, astragalus, holy basil, hawthorn, nettle, hops, and angelica to open and clear the heart chakra.

One of the best ways to take herbs is to drink them as tea. For the heart chakra, I recommend Buddha Teas' soothing and 100% organic Heart Chakra Tea which you can buy here. This tea is infused with the essence of rose *q*uartz.

Practice empathy by asking "What if?":
It can be easy for the mind to make rash conclusions about other people. Often these conclusions are judgmental, harsh, and unloving. The next time you find yourself feeling angry towards another person, ask the question "What if?" For example, if someone is rude to you, ask, "What if that person just lost their job?" Or if you struggle to get along with someone else, ask, "What if that person's childhood

traumatized them so much that they can't relate to others?" Remember that there is always a story behind the behavior of others.

Hug more:

Human beings are social creatures that require loving physical contact in order to remain healthy. Hugging releases oxytocin which is a chemical that calms down the entire body and is a natural antidepressant. Try to hug your loved ones more. If you don't have anyone to hug, try hugging yourself as an expression of self-love.

Show self-love by giving yourself the permission to feel:

One of the greatest forms of violence we show towards ourselves unknowingly is avoiding our emotions. Our emotions are not made to be controlled, repressed or shut out – they are expressions of our humanity that we need to embrace. Give yourself the permission to be unhappy, angry, sad, bored, jealousy, and all emotions which you usually shun. Anchor yourself in your breath, and allow these emotions to pass through you. Read more about opening your heart and experiencing your emotions.

Allow yourself to receive love:

Often times we tend to ignore or downplay expressions of love from other people out of low self-esteem and fear. Instead of denying affection or compliments, experiment with accepting them graciously. You might feel a little bit awkward at first, but this simple change in behavior can open up your heart more.

Meditate with the following crystals:
Use crystals as energetic totems that will help you balance your heart energy. Try meditating or carrying crystals such as jade, malachite, rose quartz, emerald, rhodonite, prehnite, ruby, green fluorite, and chrysocolla. My favorite at the moment is rhodonite.

Be thankful and show gratitude:
It's unfortunate that we take so much for granted. One of the best heart chakra healing practices out there is simply to acknowledge all the blessings you have. Simply sit down and look at, or think of, all the things you love about your life. Silently say "thank you" to each one of them or say a prayer of gratitude if that feels appropriate.

Do shadow work:
Often when our heart chakra is closed, it means that we are storing a lot of dark energy within our subconscious minds. Your shadow self is the part of you where all of your rejected and denied personality traits, thoughts, feelings, habits, and socially unacceptable ego parts are stored. When you start to access these locked away parts of you and embrace them, your heart immediately opens a little more. Read more about the shadow self and shadow work.

Do a forgiveness ritual:

Forgiveness starts with you first. In what ways have you mistreated yourself? Write a loving letter to yourself asking for forgiveness, and either burn it or keep it someplace safe. If you're holding onto resentment towards another person, try a self-designed ritual that includes one of the elements (earth, fire, water, wind). For example, if you need to forgive your mother, try lighting a candle and saying a prayer such as, "Dear Life/Spirit, may my heart release resentment towards my mother. Amen." Then blow out the candle.

Jewelry and stone for Heart chakra

The heart chakra colors test indicates that green is the color most closely associated with this chakra. Consequently, many of the following heart healing stones are green:

Jade:
This semi-precious heart chakra stone is linked to balance, and to emotional healing. You can benefit from focusing on this stone when you are dealing with a loss or an emotional injury.

Green calcite:
Traditionally used to absorb negativity, this is an excellent choice when you are finding it hard to feel empathy. This stone can help you focus on recovering from compassion fatigue.

Green aventurine:
This stone is liked to energy, vitality, and inspiration. It is said to soothe difficult emotions, and to assist in bouncing back from emotional roadblocks.

Rose quartz:
Heart chakra crystals aren't always green. This pink stone is sometimes called the "heart stone" and is said to help you regain balance.

Lifestyle and diet consideration

The best therapy for fourth chakra balance is hugging. Hugging people or pets you care about with genuine love and affection feels wonderful.

- Hugging affirms that you are loved, loving, and lovable. Even hugging yourself can be effective.

- Deep breathing is excellent for empowering both the heart and solar chakra. Cardiovascular exercise is also a great way to improve heart health, both physically and energetically.

- Buy yourself a bouquet of roses. Roses resonate at the heart chakra.

- Make yourself rosebud tea. These tiny rosebuds, which you can buy at herb shops, specialty tea shops, and at many health food stores and Asian markets, are actually a Chinese medicinal herb called mei gui hua. By steeping a few buds in a large mug of hot water for a few minutes, you can create a love ritual for yourself and ingest the love of the roses.

- Practice forgiveness—of yourself and others

Here are some of the best heart chakra foods to consume when you feel blocked or unsettled:

Green foods:
Anything green is linked to the heart chakra. This means you can't go wrong with ingredients like kale, limes, green bell peppers, spinach and green apples. All of these can help balance your heart.

Warm soups:
A hearty and rich soup can help to replenish your emotional stores and help you recover from difficult experiences. There is also anecdotal evidence that soups can promote recovery from illness, and the immune system is often at low capacity when charkas are misaligned.

Foods rich in vitamin C:
Finally, orange juice, strawberries and other fruits that contain plenty of vitamin C can help the heart chakra. You can combine these fruits with green vegetables to create a super healthy smoothie.

Mantra for Heart chakra

Singing love songs is an obvious way to incorporate sound therapy. I also like to chant HU (sounds like hue). The HU chant is almost magical in its ability to bring about feelings of balanced love and serenity.

Chapter 6

THROAT CHAKRA VISHUDDHA

Located in the region of the neck, the throat chakra or vishuddha is the fifth of your seven chakras. The Sanskrit name translates to "Especially Pure", a fitting name for this chakra, as the throat chakra is associated with speaking your authentic voice.

The energy of the throat chakra starts in the center of the neck at the level of the throat and expands through the shoulders. This chakra is the first of the higher or upper chakras on the "chakra ladder". With a strong connection to your second or sacral chakra, your throat chakra embodies your true originality and authenticity.

The throat chakra is motivated by expression and truth, it allows you to see the knowledge that is true, beyond the limitations of social conditioning. This chakra is responsible for communicating effectively and with conviction. When your fifth chakras energy is in harmony, you will stand up for what you believe in, be honest with yourself, and speak your truth.

As the center of communication and creativity, the throat chakra allows you to express who you are but also listen deeply to others. When your throat chakra is balanced, it gives you the ability to be inspired, projects your ideas, and align your vision with reality.

The throat chakra is all about speaking your truth, effectively communicating your needs, and expressing yourself. The following meditations, crystal techniques, essential oil applications, and yoga postures will help you connect with what you may be holding in this chakra, and, most importantly, initiate connection with this energy vortex within you, so that you may open into the wisdom it holds.

Identifying Blocked Throat Chakra and symptoms

Disfunctions in this energy plexus can cause disease in the related systems

- Laryngitis

- Sore throats

- Dizziness

- Asthma

- Fatigue

- Anemia

Other signs that indicate a blockage of the throat chakra are:
- Struggling to find your words or/and being afraid to talk

- Getting nervous when you find it difficult to express yourself

- Believing that it makes no sense to express yourself because most probably you will be misunderstood

- Allowing others to dominate you verbally

- Being afraid of conflicts in order to avoid controversy.

Balancing the Throat Chakra

Chakra balancing is the process of restoring the harmonious and balanced flow of prana or energy throughout the body. Your chakras are in constant fluctuation. Practicing chakra balancing and aligning is a regular and sometimes daily activity to explore. But how do you balance your throat chakra?

Use Your Voice:
As the center of your authentic voice, it is important that you practice using your voice to help restore balance to this chakra. Talking with close friends and family can be helpful. Make it a point to always speak openly and honestly with all that you say. Speaking in a heartfelt way can work wonders on your throat chakra.

Get Outside:
One of the elements that the throat chakra is influenced by is ether. Ether is the clear sky, the upper regions of air beyond the clouds. Getting outside on clear and cloudless days can help bring balance to your throat chakra. Simply taking a walk or

meditating outside on a clear day will help restore the harmonious flow of energy in your fifth chakra.

Physical Activity:
Yoga is a paramount tool in bringing balance to your throat chakra. Yoga poses for the throat chakra should focus on opening the neck and shoulders and draw energy into the throat chakra. Below are specific yoga poses and movements to connect you to the energy of the throat chakra.

Plow Pose | Halasana
Bridge Pose | Setu Bandha Sarvangasana
Child's Pose | Balasana
Upward Plank Pose | Purvottanasana

Meditation:
Sit with your shoulders back and spine straight. Relax your muscles as you close your eyes and breathe deeply. Inhale through your nose and exhale through the mouth.

Focus your attention on the location of your throat chakra: the center of the throat.

Since the throat chakra is tied to the color of blue, imagine a blue glow at the center of your throat, slowly expanding throughout your neck and shoulders, making the whole area warm and relaxed. Rest in this sensation for 3-5 minutes.

When you are ready, slowly open your eyes.

Affirmations:
Positive affirmations are a great way to heal negative programming that can be embedded in your subtle body. When balancing your throat chakra, practice saying these phrases to yourself:

- I am open and honest in my communication
- I have a right to speak my truth
- I live an authentic life
- I nourish my creativity and self-expression
- I know when to listen

Healing your Throat Chakra

Every problem has a solution and there are certainly beneficial activities that will help you unblock your throat chakra or improve its functionality:

- Warm up your voice 7 times a day with soft musical notes

- Write letters (even if you do not send them, what matters is to express yourself, put on paper everything you want to say to someone, good or bad)

- Read a text out loud

- Have a dialogue with your inner child – in writing or verbally, out loud or in your head

- Keep your palms on your ears for a few minutes

- Neck exercises such as head rotation

- Silence – Take a few moments a day where you are on your own, in silence

- Be honest! When you're afraid to express yourself, make an effort and say honestly what you have to say. Just speak from your heart and everything will be fine!

- Express your creativity! Develop your hobbies

- Respiration exercises where you deeply inhale and exhale (Try Ujjayi Breathing techniques)

- Sing as often as you can

Although there may be various reasons that could affect the throat chakra, it is recommendable to recognize the signs of blockage. You need to identify the real cause and develop a personalized set of solutions that could help you overcome the obstacles.

Yoga poses:

Easy Neck Release
To warm up the throat, start with a gentle release to soften and open your neck.
Make your way into a comfortable seated position. Place the index and middle fingers of your right hand on your left temple. Inhale deeply and draw the crown of the head toward the sky and tuck the chin into the chest.
As you exhale, tip the right ear toward your right shoulder. Use your fingers as a guide to apply gentle pressure to the temple.

Stay for 10 to 15 breaths, releasing the right shoulder down and away from the ear. To release, gently prop your head upright using your fingers. Switch sides.

2. Baby Cobra Pose
Bhujangasana

From your seated position, make your way onto your stomach. Let the chin rest on the floor and draw the big toes together. Place the arms under the shoulder blades and tuck your elbows tightly in by your ribs.

On an inhale, lift the head and chest from the mat and gaze softly a few inches in front of your hands. Feel the abdominal muscle engage against the floor as the neck opens. Keep the elbows tucked tightly against the ribs to work the biceps. As you exhale, lower the head and chest and rest the chin on the floor.

If you want to open the neck further, lift the head and chest higher and let the bottom ribs graze the floor to explore the full expression of Cobra Pose, straightening through your elbow. Be mindful of any strain on your low back.

Complete up to 5 reps and roll over onto your back.

3. Supported Fish Pose
Matsyasana

Supported Fish Pose can make you feel uncomfortable and vulnerable. Breathe into the sensations, letting the neck and shoulders release as the throat and heart begin to open up.

Place a block between your shoulder blades. Lower the mid-back over the block (at the back of your heart) and let the head and neck release down toward the floor, opening the throat to the sky.

Find a comfortable leg position, such as stretching the legs long or bending the knees and placing the feet on the floor.

If you don't have a block, using a small pillow or rolled-up blanket. Stay for at least 10-15 breaths.

4. Shoulder Stand

Salamba Sarvangasana

Shoulder Stand is a great counter-pose for the back and shoulders after coming out of Fish Pose. This inversion reverses circulation and sends fresh blood to the throat.

Lie flat on your back with your arms and legs extended. Lift your legs into the air and flex the feet flat like you're going to talk a walk on the ceiling. Roll the torso up and off of the mat to take the weight of the legs and torso onto your shoulders. Use your arms and hands as kickstands to support your lower back.

Stay for 5-10 breaths.

5. Legs-Up-The-Wall Pose

Viparita Kirani

If Shoulder Stand is not in your practice, try Legs up the Wall for a modified inversion.

Lie next to a wall on the floor or bed and extend the legs skyward, flexing the feet flat. Stay for 5-10 breaths before gently releasing into Savasana to rest for a few minutes.

Jewelry and stone for Throat Chakra

Each chakra is influenced by unique stones and their energetic properties. The throat chakra is highly influenced by lapis lazuli. When balancing your throat chakra, meditate with lapis lazuli, carry the stone with you, or wear jewelry with lapis lazuli to let the energetic properties help restore balance to the chakra. Our Throat Chakra Blend has a lapis lazuli rollerball to aid in balancing your throat chakra. Lapis Lazuli Rollerball: Known as the stone of truth, lapis lazuli is used to open and balance the throat chakra. The elements of lapis lazuli stimulate the desire for knowledge, truth, and understanding. The energetic properties of lapis lazuli restore your ability to communicate and speak your truth.

Lifestyle and diet consideration

Balance your fifth chakra with blue foods. Blueberries and blackberries are particularly good sources of fiber, antioxidants, and vitamins. For the throat chakra, think healing and soothing foods and liquids such as coconut water, herbal teas, raw honey, and lemon. Fruit that grows on trees such as apples, pears, and plums are also known to be excellent at healing this chakra.

Make This: Homemade Elderflower Syrup
Wear This: Turquoise

Mantra for Throat chakra

"HUM" is Mantra sound for throat chakra.

Chapter 7

THIRD EYE CHAKRA AJNA

Third Eye Chakra, is sometimes referred to as the Brow Chakra, is the sixth chakra. Energetically the sacral chakra vibrates to the color Indigo. Your third eye chakra is an energy center in the middle of your brow. This energy center, also called the sixth, brow and ajna chakra, represents your insight, intuition, and intelligence. It also relates to psychic awareness, sometimes referred to as the sixth sense. Lucid dreams and dream recall are components of the third eye energy center. This chakra embodies the purposeful use of imagination. The Third eye chakra is located at the base of the skull at the medulla oblongata and is between the two physical eyes and in the middle of the head. The third eye governs the pineal gland, pituitary glands, brain, eyes, ears, nose. It also governs the sinuses.

The third eye is the chakra of wisdom—enough to see, and the intellect to understand both sides of every event or story. Here we find our mystical selves—intuition, inner vision, a deeper perception of life than before. This is the place of shamans and wisdom keepers, those whose introspection open the doors of past lives, subconscious pattern recognition, astral travel, and extrasensory perception.

This is the chakra of dreams that provide information to guide us, and that of remembering them when we wake. The pineal gland secretes serotonin which regulates sleep patterns and melatonin which may be responsible for our circadian rhythms.

When you balance the third eye chakra, you experience clarity of thought and vision, you are imaginative, intuitive, and see the events in your life as symbolic and lessons to be learned. You will remember your dreams and contemplate their meanings. You are flexible in your opinions. Those who balance the third eye often become visionaries, often telepathic, and are not afraid of death because, to them, it is merely an extension of life in a different realm.

As with the other chakras, however, imbalances occur and come in either excess or as deficiencies. When out of balance, you might experience headaches, problems with the eyes and/or ears, sleep disorders or anxiety related issues. Those who are in balance, or nearly there, cannot tolerate negative or violent environments, or what they see that does not correspond with what they have heard about a situation.

Identifying Blocked Third eye Chakra and symptoms

- inability to plan or set goals

- narrow-minded

- denial

- poor vision/memory

- difficulty seeing future

- lack of imagination

Balancing the Third Eye Chakra

Meditation, especially with an open third eye, is always a good place to start and a critical component to balance the third eye. Meditating under natural light is most beneficial and a good place to start, either sunlight or moonlight. (During the winter you can substitute with full spectrum light.)

Concentrate on breathing. With your eyes closed "look" at the area between your eyebrows. This may take several to many attempts, especially if you've never attempted to open your third eye. You might try thinking of the color purple and trying to "see" it between your eyebrows (your third eye). Be patient, with enough time and work, your third eye will open.

When I want to balance all my chakras, I start trying to "see" red, then orange, yellow, green, blue, purple and finally white. If you have trouble, think of Santa Claus for red, and orange to eat, a yellow flower, etc. as you go through them.

Sleep is another critical component of third eye balance. Be sure you get enough sleep at night which should be seven to eight hours. The time between 1:00 and 4:00 a.m. are important for this chakra; the ancients felt this was the when we connected with our higher beings. If you have sleep problems, try breathing exercises or a CD with a guided meditation. Put your "screens" away at least an hour before you go to bed. If you like to read, you'll need to put the Kindle or Nook away and read an actual paper book! Try not eating for at least two or three hours before bedtime. Art therapy is another way to induce sleep, or self-hypnosis if you are able.

Aromatherapy:

The following are essential oils to consider as aromatherapy. These essential oils can be diluted to 3% in a carrier oil on your pulse points, or on a cotton ball or in a diffuser for inhalation.

Aromatherapy to balance the Third Eye:

- Frankincense (Boswellia carteri)

- Lavender (Lavandula angustifolia)

- Neroli (Citrus x aurantium)

- Juniper (Juniperus communis)

- Diffusing lavender at bedtime is helpful and calming.

Healing your Third Eye chakra

Use a daily affirmation:
designed to activate your third eye. Try, 'I am a wise decision maker,' 'I am open to the wisdom within,' 'I trust my intuition.'

Practice dialoging with the Divine:
Ask a question and then relax into waiting for a response. Remember the Divine speaks to us in messages, signs, and symbols. Be prepared to wait and be open to receiving information in any form.

Keep a dream journal:
Write down whatever fragments you remember first thing each morning, before putting your feet to the floor.

Go star gazing.

Also you can:

1) Use healing stones that have the same vibrational frequency as the third eye. Good examples are purple fluorite, lapis lazuli, moonstone, amethyst, and quartz.

2) Dark blue or purple foods will have a positive effect on the third eye. Eat more plums, eggplant, cabbage, kale, blueberries, and purple peppers. Foods naturally rich in Omega-3's (brain food) are also good.

Remember to give time to balancing your entire chakra system – particularly the root chakra. An overall balanced system makes it much easy to work with one or two chakras that are particularly blocked.

3) Find an art form that you enjoy, or think you might enjoy, and engage in it regularly. Creating art stimulates both the third eye and crown chakras.

4) Visualize the color indigo between your eyes during meditation. Hold the color there for 5-10 minutes

5) Detoxify your pineal gland by eliminating chemicals like fluoride, alcohol, pesticides. Also, make sure you're drinking plenty of water... And eating an abundance of dark leafy greens like spinach, chard, spirulina, and kale.

6) Consider both acupuncture and acupressure as additions to your physical health regimens.

7) Drop down into your body. If you feel that your mind is racing, an indication of an overactive third eye, do some grounding work and body awareness work to help calm you down.

8) Connect with the element of light by finding the broadest expanse of blue sky, lying down, and then just relaxing.

9) Find a non-competitive exercise to practice regularly.

10) Practice opening up to your intuition by setting an intention each morning to pay attention and act on intuitive signals.

11) Make time to be in silence and solitude on a regular, if not daily basis. Five to ten minutes a day are all that are required. Put away all electronic devices and sit or lie in silence, paying attention to internal sensations and cues.

Yoga practices for third eye:

Candle Gazing (Trataka)
This practice connects you with the energy of the Third Eye Chakra by stimulating your two eyes and encouraging a deep state of focus using the image of a dancing flame.
Sit comfortably. Place a candle before you at a distance where you can gaze at the flame with an upright head and neck. Gaze intensely until your eyes water a bit and then let your eyelids almost close. In the gap, focus on the glow of the flame. Finally, close your eyelids completely and focus on the afterglow that remains. It will often look like a small purple or

red dot that dances across the darkness of your closed eyelids.

Try to maintain this practice for two to three minutes..

Wide-Legged Forward Fold (Prasarita Padottanasana)

There's nothing like turning upside down to change your perspective. This accessible inverted posture brings your head below your heart and provides a powerful shift for your perception.

Face the long edge of your mat and walk your feet apart from each other as far as you comfortably can. Inhale and either hold a belt or towel behind your back or interlace your fingers behind you. With an elongated spine, exhale and hinge forward from your hips.

Let your forehead come into contact with a block, a stack of books, or the surface of a chair or sofa. No need to strain your legs and back trying to reach down to a level that is uncomfortable.

Stay here for one to two minutes. Come out of the pose by bending your knees and extending your spine long to rise up to standing with an elongated back.

Nadi Shodhana Pranayama (Alternate Nostril Breathing)

This powerful breathing technique brings balance to the right and left hemispheres of your brain by harmonizing the energy flowing toward the "rational" left brain and the "intuitive" right brain.

Find a comfortable seat and take a few natural breaths. When you are ready to proceed, raise your right hand and rest your index finger and middle finger on your forehead at your Third Eye Chakra.Let your thumb rest on your right nostril. Rest your ring finger and little finger on your left nostril. Block your right nostril with your thumb and inhale through your left nostril.

Next, block your left nostril and release your thumb to exhale through your right nostril. Alternate this pattern of breathing from left to right and then right to left 10 to 15 times.If you prefer to visualize your breath moving in this pattern, it is possible to do this technique with your hands resting in your lap. In this version, imagine that your breath has a color and watch it make the shape of an inverted "V" that rises up the length of one nostril to the Third Eye Chakra and down the length of the opposite nostril to leave the body.

To close the practice, take three to four neutral and natural breaths through both nostrils.

Jewelry and stone for Third Eye chakra

The thought is that you can find jewelry featuring purple stones and wear it anytime you need to unblock the third eye chakra. You can also purchase larger third eye crystals that will sit in your pocket or in the palm of your hand, allowing you to squeeze them and focus on them when you need to keep your third eye chakra open. Some of the best third eye stones include the following:

Purple fluorite: This semi-precious gem is supposed to promote sharpened intuition and to clear up muddled thoughts. It's an ideal third eye chakra crystal when you're trying to make a difficult choice and want to

get rid of irrelevant distractions.

Amethyst: A famous and beautiful precious stone, amethyst is traditionally connected to third eye headache relief as well as all forms of healing. Some people also use it to represent wisdom.

Black Obsidian: Another popular member of the third eye crystals group, black obsidian promotes balance between emotion and reason.

Lifestyle and diet consideration

As is intuitive, basic chakra foods (i.e. ones that help all chakras) are all healthy staples. For example, all fruits, vegetables, healthy fats and wholegrain foods tend to promote openness throughout the chakra system. Eat foods such as black currants, blueberries, blackberries, eggplant, prunes, beets, and rainbow chard. Remove fluoride from your diet using a water purifying system because fluoride calcifies the pineal gland, which is directly linked to the third eye chakra. However, there are also specific third eye chakra foods, and adding them to your daily diet can help to prevent or combat blockages. Keep the following in mind:

Dark chocolate:
If you like dark chocolate, feel free to have as much as you want when you're trying to open the third eye! It is said to help enhance mental clarity and boost concentration. It is a great source of magnesium, which destresses you. As a bonus, it promotes the release of serotonin, putting you in a more positive mood.

Anything purple:
Given that purple is the third eye's color, all purple foods promote its balance. Some of the best examples include eggplant, purple cabbage, red grapes, blueberries, and blackberries.

Omega-3: Foods that are rich in omega-3 can enhance cognitive function and thereby help to keep your third eye chakra open. Good choices include walnuts, salmon, chia seeds and sardines.

Wear This: Howlite or Quartz

Lifestyle Also Include:

- When you receive an intuitive hint, act on it.

- It will strengthen your intuition.

- Set the intention that you wish to connect with your inner wisdom.

- Add dark blue and indigo colors to your wardrobe.

Mantra for Third Eye chakra

Chant the sound "SHAM."

Chapter 8

CROWN CHAKRA SAHASRARA

The crown chakra is all about becoming more connected with our Inner Divine, as well as our connection to the Divine. The following meditations, crystal techniques, essential oil applications, and yoga postures will help you connect with what you may be holding in this chakra. Most importantly, these techniques will help you initiate connection with this energy vortex within you so you may open into the wisdom it holds.

Symptoms of blockage of the Crown Chakra: From a physiological point of view, a blocked Sahasrara manifests through headaches, migraines, weak memory, nervous system imbalances, poor coordination, fatigue, low vision and sore throat or ear tingling. However, it is important to remember that in some cases, these symptoms may be caused by other factors and are not always the effect of a dysfunctional crown chakra. For this reason, it is recommendable to seek medical advice.

On the other hand, the emotional aspect of one's life is also profoundly affected by a flawed crown chakra. The common symptoms are sadness or anxiety episodes without any obvious reason, lack of desire to communicate and stubborn rejection of the ideas of others.

Moreover, one does not get involved in the lives of loved ones and often feels s/he is a spectator of their own life where things are done without control and direction. These often lead to isolation and a sense of spiritual disconnection.

Identifying Blocked Crown Chakra and symptoms

Shallow Relationships:

The fear of being socially isolated drives many of us to accept people in our lives that may not be beneficial to our spiritual growth. Thus, we lower our standards and change our perspectives on life. As a result, we tolerate behaviors that do not match our personality in order to maintain a connection with the people around us.

This should change. If you are surrounded by selfish and toxic people who seem to leave you emotionally drained, then it is more likely that they are an obstacle to your spiritual growth.

Fear of Change:

Change equals challenge and a step out of the comfort zone. It challenges our barriers and promotes our growth, even though the process may cause discomfort or fear.

Whatever may worry you, you should discover ways that will help you evolve and overcome fear.

Repressed Emotions:
The modern society continues motivating us to adopt a positive thinking and approach when facing challenges or dealing with people of a different character. Although this is highly essential in keeping a balanced spiritual energy, we often forget that sadness and anger are normal feelings too.

We often tend to think that being overly critical or making negative remarks are signs of a problematic soul with limited understanding. In reality, repressing emotions can have severe effects on your emotional and mental well-being, leaving you depressed, angry and unhappy.

Ego:
Our spirit is in continuous search for fulfillment, wishing to serve its purpose and give love, care and kindness.

On the other hand, our ego strives for earthly conditions and rewards, such as luxury, social affirmation, personal style, or attention. A life filled with these materialistic and selfish matters give us only a temporary relief. We ignore and block our soul's desire of expressing its needs or fulfill its purpose.

Balancing Your Crown chakra

An imbalanced crown chakra can also manifest itself in many ways. Living in a state of constant worry, headaches, general lack of purpose, depression and an inability to connect with your higher wisdom are only a few ways that an unhealthy crown chakra can be displayed. So let's learn five ways to cleanse and balance your crown chakra.

Meditate:
Your crown chakra is strongly affected by meditation, as it's your connection to your higher self and the higher power that you believe in. Imagine a golden light illuminating the entire crown of your head, including the space a little bit above your head. It helps me to think of the halos depicted in religious imagery. Feel this glow illuminate and recharge not only your physical body, but your spirit as well. Allow this soft yet powerful light to reconnect you with the world around you—and to your own authentic self, your own true light.

Check your ego:
Self-confidence and ego are not the same. Learning to let go of your ego-driven life will benefit you in many ways, not the least of which is a much healthier crown chakra. One thing to consider is that ego is often fueled by insecurity, but true confidence comes from real self-knowledge—and acceptance.

Choose love:
You can't fully love another until you love yourself is a frustratingly true statement, and learning to love yourself for who you already are is also the first step towards accepting others. So choose love, and as an added bonus you'll likely let go of tension from your other chakras as well.

Prayer:
Prayer is a very personal thing for many people, but it doesn't have to be formal or foreign. Prayer can be as simple as setting an intention in your daily yoga practice. So close your eyes and let the voice of the deeper you be your guide.

Finding your innermost self is, for most of us, a lifelong journey. Learning to tap into the stillness that's always present underneath the currents of daily life is a great place to begin making this connection, and this new-found self-awareness and love will hopefully be just the beginning of a healthy relationship with so much more.

Healing Your Crown Chakra

We now know what obstacles may prevent a proper functioning of the crown chakra. Let's explore the steps we should take to heal our spiritual energy:

Reconnect with Yourself:
Define what you need in your life, listen to your soul's needs and your intuition will guide you. But in order to hear your inner voice clearer, you should remove all the negativity around you. It may be coming from toxic relationships, stressful career, unspoken thoughts or repressed emotions.
Another option would be to focus on your hobbies as they can be great healing methods.

Surround yourself with beauty:
Whether it is music, nature or art, you should nurture your soul with objects that do not reflect the materialistic world we live in today.
Have longer walks in nature or listen to classical music that brings you tranquility and helps you reconnect with yourself.

Do kind acts:
Scientifically speaking, researchers found that 95% of people who do random acts of kindness feel happier with themselves and more optimistic about life.

Moreover, they also have a lower blood pressure and less anxiety!

Why is that? We are created to care for one another and the unhappiness of others becomes our unhappiness.

Dedicate time to spiritual dimension:

Since we are talking about a spiritual chakra, perhaps the most effective way to equilibrate its energy is to pray or meditate (depending on your spiritual beliefs).

In the end, our spirit's goal is to remain connected to the Higher Energy. We can make that happen through prayers, reflective thinking and meditation such as yoga or reiki.

Yoga poses:

Ardha Padmasana or Half Lotus Pose

How to: Start by sitting in an easy pose (sukhasana) on the mat. For further support, beginners can sit on a cushion to stay longer in the pose. Lift the left foot and gently place it on the right thigh, while the other foot stays underneath the left thigh.

Place the hands on the knees. Stay here and mediate if you can hold for long enough or practice daily to achieve the long duration required for mediation.

Why to: Lotus pose or Padamasana is one of the most opted poses for meditation as it neutralises blood pressure, balances the body and calms the mind. Directly tapping into the higher consciousness, half lotus pose extend the same benefits as a full lotus pose and is a great practice for beginners.

Vriksasana or Tree Pose

How to: Start with Mountain pose, keep the feet hip width apart. Extend your spine tall and fix your gaze forward at a focal point. Breathe in and lift the right leg and place the sole of your right foot on the left leg, inner thigh. The heel of the right leg should touch the perineum otherwise, can rest on the thigh, or even on the calf initially.

Lifting the torso upwards, take a deep breath & raise the arms up, joining the hands in Namaste mudra. If you can, take your gaze upwards towards the ceiling. Stay here for 5 to 7 breaths and repeat on the other side.

Why to: A restorative and a balancing pose, the position of the arms and gaze taps into the energies of the crown chakra. The position of the body, works from root to the tip of the head, by aligning the chakras in a string. Also, rejuvenating the mind, it strengths the whole body.

Savasana or Corpse Pose

How to: Lie gently on your back, lift your pelvis and slide your tailbone away to comfortably spread your lower back. Keep just a light, natural arch to your lower back. Rest your pelvis on the ground. Place both the feet and the arms 3 to 4 feet apart with palms facing the ceiling. Support the back of the head and neck on a folded blanket, if you like.

Now close your eyes and take a slow deep breath. As you exhale, let your body relax and sink into the floor.

Maintain stillness as you relax and *q*uiet the mind. Loosen your whole body completely, like its sinking in the floor. Stay here for as long as you like.

Why to: This pose gets its name from the posture of a dead body. It re*q*uires the stillness of a corpse, which makes it a challenging one. It helps in the repair of tissues and cells and in releasing stress. Savasana helps to calm and balance the crown chakra.

Salamba Sirsasana or Supported Headstand

How to: An advance pose, Supported Headstand can be performed by following a series of preparatory postures. An expert's guiding presence is recommended initially.

Come in Dolphin pose and place the head in between your elbows, like your hands are cupping the tip of the head. Inhale and reach up through the balls of your feet until your body form a V, thereby raising the hips to the ceiling. The majority of the weight would have shifted to your forearms and shoulders by now. Start by lifting one leg, feet pointing upwards.

Keep the abdomen tight. Stay here for a couple of breaths and try the other leg. Keep practicing this position for a couple of days till you get a hang of the weight on the shoulders and head.

Use the abdominal muscles to raise both feet up together and draw the thighs in the abdomen. The torso should remain perpendicular to the floor. Exhale and lift the legs gently towards the ceiling.

Keep the weight evenly balanced on the two forearms. The whole procedure can be first practiced against the wall, in order to avoid any injury and gradually once you build strength you can move away from the wall.

Why to: This pose inverts the flow of the blood completely towards the head, giving rest to all the organs in the body. In Headstand, the crown of your head is on the floor, which means it is grounded and connected to the earth. An effective and a sure shot way to create awareness and balance in the crown area, this pose will restore the flow of energy in your body.

Nadi Shodhan Pranayama or Alternate Nostril Breathing

How to: Connected to the two hemispheres of the brain, our nostrils are gateways to reservoir of charged energies. This breathing practice or Pranayama balances and activates the Ida and Pingala Nadis. Sit in an easy pose and start by forming a Nasika Mudra, i.e. First two fingers folded and last two fingers and thumb stretched out.

Place the thumb on the right nostril, and inhale from the left nostril, hold your breath for 2-3 seconds. Now close the left nostril with the last two fingers and exhale from the right nostril. Again, inhale from the right, close the right nostril with the thumb and then exhale from the left. Repeat the procedure for 5 to 7 times on each side.

Why to: Nadi Shodhana pranayama helps to bring the mind back to the present moment and is an excellent breathing technique to calm and center the mind. It regulates the breath, increases the psychic abilities of the practitioner, and also balances both the hemispheres of the brain.

Other advance poses that activates and stimulate the crown chakra are Wheel Pose or Chakra Asana, Hand Stand, Crane Pose or Bakasana, Lotus Pose or Padamasana; King Pigeon Pose.

Jewelry and stone for Crown chakra

Crown Chakra jewelry collection is made with Amethyst and Purple Agate gemstones that represent and energize your center of consciousness and spiritual awareness, also known as Sahasrana. The crown chakra is also known as the Seventh chakra, it's located above your head, and it's represented by the color violet or purple, which acts as a protector to people seeking to live a more spiritual life. Wear Crown Chakra jewelry to help in your connection to a higher power and spiritual growth.

Lifestyle and diet consideration

The best lifestyle habit for crown health is prayer or meditation. Prayer is simply expressing your inner thoughts about life and asking for guidance. Meditation reduces mental clutter and allows you to follow inspirations when they come. I believe that meditation is the best thing you can do for achieving both a meaningful life and a healthy and balanced crown chakra.

The crown chakra focuses more on fasting and detoxing than it does on food. It focuses more on the spiritual aspect of our bodies; our minds. Detoxing can help our bodies flush out toxins, boost our energy, and clear our mind. Meditation and yoga is an excellent way to strengthen and heal the crown chakra. It can teach us to live mindfully and take some *q*uiet, peaceful time for ourselves amidst our chaotic lives. Meditation herbs or essential oils such as sage, lavender, frankincense, and juniper are wonderful in balancing this chakra.

Mantra for Crown chakra

The mantra for your crown is "ALL". For the crown energy center, chant all in a row, "LAM, VAM, RAM, YAM, HAM, OM, ALL" in one breath, inhale, and repeat as many times as I care to, usually a total of 7 times. The first five mantra sounds all rhyme with "mom"!

Chapter 9

Chakra Meditations

The Science Behind Chakra

Chakra meditation is a powerful form of spiritual enlightenment which focuses on the 7 specific energy points in the body. Each energy point relates to certain aspects of our lives which can be enhanced and improved through meditation.

Whether you realize it or not, your Chakras are at work within your body constantly. They influence your mental as well as your physical state. By paying special attention to these areas, you can influence them to improve certain aspects of your life. As already discussed above, let us take have an overview at each of the 7 Chakras in detail and which areas of your body and life they can influence:

The Root Chakra: This is the first Chakra, located at the very base of the spine. It symbolizes the energy of the earth flowing into the body and is the correlation between our physical presence and the material world. The colour synonymous with the Root Chakra is red and it is associated with health, protection and well-being. Meditating on this Chakra or the colour red will enhance these areas in your life.

The Sacral Chakra: This Chakra is located just above the Root Chakra, in the lower part of the abdomen. It signifies energies associated with sexuality, happiness, love, compassion, sympathy and understanding. Its corresponding colour is orange. Feelings associated with giving and receiving are tied to this Chakra. Meditating on this Chakra or the colour orange will allow you to control emotions.

The Solar Plexus Chakra: Located above the Naval Chakra just below the chest, this point focuses on willpower and self-transformation. The power of the subconscious mind, discipline of the ego and ability to control one's self all emanate from this Chakra, which is associated with the colour yellow. Meditate on this one to control your external circumstances as well as your self esteem.

The Heart Chakra: Associated with the colour green, it signifies energy associated with kind nature, forgiveness and unconditional love which extends beyond the physical realm. This Chakra is located in the middle of the chest and centres around perseverance, harmony and patience. Meditating on this Chakra will allow you to heal pain through the power of love.

The Throat Chakra: Located just below the chin in the throat. It symbolizes the power of all forms of communication and how *q*ualities like truth, nobility, character and wisdom can be conveyed with the correct purpose and respect. It is associated with the colour sky blue and also revolves around extra sensory communication. Meditating on this Chakra will allow you to express yourself truthfully at all times.

The Third Eye Chakra: Symbolizes intuition, insight, instinct and how the mind perceives the soul. Concentrating on this Chakra will give you peace of mind and stimulate your imagination. The colour synonymous with this Chakra is indigo and relates to spiritual guidance and direction. Meditating on it will allow you to access the path to your inner wisdom.

The Crown Chakra: The northern most Chakra in the body, located at the top of the head. It signifies the relationship between the conscious mind and its surroundings. The highest powers of the mind and spirit can be reached by meditating on this Chakra. Its associated colour is violet and it also serves to encompass the entire body within the realms of spirituality.

By concentrating on each of these Chakras in turn, great strides can be made towards empowering yourself with the ability to control the physical and non-physical elements of the body. All of the Chakras absorb and emanate energy. Meditation is the process by which this transference of energy takes place.

When all 7 Chakras have been energized, the body and the mind become one. This is when they can be most influenced to enhance or improve your life, by thinking and meditating on positive outcomes.

Master your inner self through understanding your Chakras, concentrating on each one. Starting with the Root, work your way upwards. Using this form of meditation regularly will help you understand yourself and give your life purpose.

How Chakra meditation works

Chakra meditation uses the power of your mind and your ability to visualize to change your energy. Your mind can affect energy.

Chakra meditation helps you to keep your mind focused and leads you through each chakra. You are guided to perceive each chakra in the meditation.

Sometimes I have students who have trouble seeing or are still working on opening up their clairvoyance skills. This is okay if you can't actually see your chakras psychically.

You don't need to in order to have chakra meditation be effective for you. In these cases, I ask my students to feel, imagine what they think their chakras look like, or just know what that particular chakra is like.

However you perceive is fine. It's the intention and the focus that are important in clearing your chakras.

If you find there is one particular chakra that is harder to visualize or takes longer to clear, it means that there a particular resistance in the energy field. Sometimes it's a belief about ourselves or the world that we hold to stubbornly. Other times it's because we habitually neglect our own needs of rest and relaxation.

If you have trouble visualizing the colour, you might want to pick up some bright paint chips, one for each chakra colour and have it with you for the chakra meditation. You can use them as reference as you need to.

Root Chakra Meditation

This meditation activates the first chakra center and is strongly grounding to the mind and emotions. Sit in a comfortable position, either cross-legged on the floor or in a chair. Sit up tall with the spine straight, the shoulders relaxed and the chest open. Rest the hands on your knees or in your lap with the palms facing up. Relax the face, jaw, and belly. Let the tongue rest on the roof of the mouth, just behind the front teeth. Allow the eyes to lightly close. Breathe slowly, smoothly and deeply in and out through the nose. Breathe deeply down into the low belly, all the way down to the perineum. Bring your awareness to the 1st chakra, Muladhara, located between the tip of the tailbone and the bottom of the pubic bone. Notice any sensations here as you take a few slow deep breaths in and out. Then inhale and engage Mula Bandha by contracting the muscles between the pubic bone and tailbone and drawing the perineum up towards Muladhara. Keep your focus on feeling Mula Bandha and Muladhara as the breath flows in and the muscles contract. Feel the spine lengthen up as the feet and legs ground down. If comfortable, hold the breath in for 1-2 seconds. Then release Mula Bandha and exhale the air out through the nose. Repeat for 3-5 minutes, working on increasing the contraction of Mula Bandha if comfortable. Return to a slow deep breath with awareness of Muladhara without engaging Mula Bandha. Feel any sensations here as you take a few slow deep breaths in and out, noticing any changes. Breathe deeply into Muladhara for 3-5 minutes. To end, gently let the eyes blink open, inhale the palms together in front of the heart, exhale and gently bow. Take a moment or two before moving on with the rest of your day.

Sacral Chakra Meditation

Sit in a comfortable cross-legged position with your spine straight, or lie down in Savasana, Corpse Pose. Take a few deep breaths through the nose to center yourself and to start calming the mind. Bring your awareness to pelvic area and imagine a ball of bright orange light there. Keep breathing deeply and steadily through the nose. Visualise the ball of orange light growing, expanding and strengthening with each inhale. You may feel the orange energy swirling clockwise and you may experience warmth or tingling in the pelvis and/or lower back. Keep breathing. Maintain your awareness on the energy and keep working on expanding it, for as long as you can. When you wish to come out of the meditation, give gratitude for the experience and resume your day.

Solar plexus chakra meditation

Begin with several minutes of deep breathing, and then once you're suitably relaxed and focused you can move onto a visualization stage that helps you access the solar plexus chakra: Turn your attention to your upper abdomen, where the solar plexus chakra resides. Picture a round sphere of glowing yellow light in the center of the upper abdomen, and slowly concentrate on making the energy wider and brighter. Imagine the sphere rotating (clockwise) as it grows, and feel the area becoming warmer and more relaxed as you do this. After 3-5 minutes, let the energy dissipate throughout your body, take a few deep breaths again and open your eyes.

Heart chakra meditation

Find a comfortable, relaxing place where you won't be disturbed. Sit and breathe in through your nose and out through your mouth for a few minutes. Feel your body relaxing as you do this. Imagine that you're drawing green energy up through your body towards the heart, starting at the base of the spine and moving upwards. Picture that energy solidifying into a bright ball of green energy sitting at the level of the heart chakra. As you inhale and exhale, see that ball becoming bigger and brighter. Focus on tuning into feelings of love for yourself and others, letting the green energy radiate through your whole body. Emerge from the meditation after 3-5 minutes.

Throat Chakra Meditation

This meditation is called Bramahri and you hum like a bee! It calms the mind, it cleanses, opens and heals the throat chakra. It also creates a pleasant and healing vibration in the body and promotes blood flow to the brain. Sit in a comfortable cross-legged position (or on a chair) with your spine straight. Place your palms on your knees. Close your eyes and start turning your attention inwards. Take a few deep breaths in and out through the nose to center yourself and to calm the mind. Bring your awareness to the breath, to its natural rhythm. Keep the eyes closed and bring the index fingers on the cartilage of the ear (between the cheek and inner ear). Take a deep breath in and as you breathe out, press very gently on the cartilage while making a loud humming sound like a bee. Repeat until you feel a vibration building up in your throat and skull. Eventually, you will feel the vibration in your whole body. Release your hands to your knees, maintain the eyes closed a little longer and notice the effects of this breathing practice on your physical, mental and emotional body. Exploring yoga poses to soothe and open the throat is integral to my personal yoga practice and my teaching. Giving your throat and neck a little extra love, help balance energy in communication, self-expression and creativity.

Third eye Chakra Meditation

Sit comfortably and close your eyes. Inhale and exhale ten times, slowly and deeply. Focus your attention on the location of the third eye chakra, imagine a violet sphere of energy in the middle of your forehead. Remember, purple is the third eye chakra's color. As you continue to breathe slowly and deeply, picture the purple ball of energy getting bigger and warmer. As it does, imagine it purging negativity from your body. Think of yourself of absorbing the third eye chakra's energy—allow yourself to feel it all over. Open your eyes when you feel ready. As you may have guessed, yoga can also be helpful when learning how to balance your chakras. Third eye yoga poses include the child pose and the eagle pose. You can find pictures and videos that will guide you through these straightforward positions. You may notice 3rd eye chakra opening symptoms soon after!

Crown Chakra Meditation

Sit in a comfortable meditation pose with your legs crossed and your back straight. If working in a group, sit in a circle. Rest your hands in your lap, palms upward, with your left hand on top. This is the mudra (hand position) for receiving energy. Close your eyes and let your breathing become slow and even. Visualize a thousand-petalled lotus at the crown of your head. Imagine its petals gently opening to reveal an intense light. Let this divine light flow down into you through your crown chakra. Repeat one of the affirmations below, or create one that has more meaning for you. If you are alone, say the words silently; in a group, you may wish to chant them out loud, in unison:

"I am surrounded and protected by divine light."

"This light nourishes my entire being."

"I am forever walking in the light."

"I grow stronger by tuning into the divine light."

Feel the light spiraling down your body. Enjoy the warm glow as it saturates your entire being. Let every cell be permeated by light and inspiration, and every part of your consciousness become illuminated. Focus your senses on the intensity of the light so that you not only see it, but hear, smell, taste, and touch it. Think of the light as a manifestation of your higher self, representing the peace that lies beyond understanding.

Feel like a pure channel for the light: allow yourself to be at one with it. In this state of oneness, intuitive thoughts and inspirations may enter your consciousness. Be thankful for this guidance. After 15 minutes, take a few deep breaths and open your eyes.

Chapter 10

How to maintain harmony and balance in your chakra

1. Spend time in nature.

Sitting in the grass or walking barefoot is a great way to feel more connected and absorb the healing energy of nature. This will also help to keep you grounded and bring more peace into your life.
Even adding flowers or plants to your home will make a positive difference.

2. Practice creative visualization.

Clearing your mind from negative chatter is the first step to successful visualization. Once your mind is clear, try visualizing images that represent happiness or love.
For example, you could visualize a flower opening or a heart blessing each of your chakras.

3. Breathe deeply.

Breathing with intention is one of the easiest and most effective ways to restore your chakras.
To help bring your chakras into their natural and harmonic balance, every time you inhale, direct the

energy of your breath to your chakra; exhale and allow awareness to settle into the chakra.

4. We are the right colors

Did you know that each of your chakras emits a different color? And each color represents a specific vibration?

Red color represents your root chakra, orange — your sacral chakra, yellow — solar plexus chakra, green or pink — heart chakra, blue — throat chakra, indigo or purple — third eye chakra, and purple or white represents your crown chakra.

So if you're working on balancing the heart chakra, for example, make sure you wear green or burn a pink candle.

5. Practice gratitude

By now, you probably know that when you're in a state of gratitude, you instantly raise your vibrational frequency.

When you raise your vibration, you open your chakras and you start attracting more positive things in your life, like abundance, happiness, peace and even better relationships!

And speaking of relationships and manifesting more success... I have a really cool surprise for you that can help you become more well-liked, confident and respected.

Making friends or connecting with people can be intimidating, especially if you're naturally shy.
And unfortunately, this can become a problem not only in your social or romantic life, but also in your career's success as well.

How to perform your chakra meditation

Because your chakras are part of an intimately connected system, there is only so much work you can do on singular chakras. It's better to meditate on all of them to bring the entire system into balance. With time and experience, you'll get better at detecting individual imbalances and directing your meditation to focus on particular chakras.

To get started, all you need to do is find a peaceful place where you won't be disturbed for at least a half hour.

Sit comfortably on the floor with your legs folded in front of you. You can sit on a cushion if you find the position uncomfortable. Hold your spine erect but not stressed. Let your hands fall limp on your knees. Breathe deeply and evenly.

What you can do is visualize each chakra in turn, from the root to the crown. As you do, you should picture the energy flowing into and through that chakra. Use the color associations of each chakra provided above during your meditation.

Give each chakra patient attention and focus on it until you can see vibrant energy passing through it. Each chakra deserves several minutes for itself.

By the time you reach the crown chakra, you should have a clear mental image of positive energy flowing all the way through your body.

When you're first starting to explore chakra meditation, it can be tricky to keep track of the energy centers and colors you need to focus on. Guided meditation tools can be an enormous help here.

These are images, videos, or audio tracks (using the mantras listed above) that help you pace your meditation and keep you focused on the proper chakra.

Individual Chakra Meditation:

After you've successfully gone through a few meditation sessions, you should start to feel more sensitized to the energy flowing through your chakras. You'll start to tie your feelings and physical state into specific chakras. Now you may want to start concentrating your sessions on individual chakras.

Do not force this process; with experience, you should find it more or less natural for your focus to drift to the chakras that are most in need of balancing when you meditate. You'll find that there are many specialized positions, breathing exercises, mantras, and gestures (mudras) available to help you concentrate on specific chakras.

Chapter 1

Spirituality and connection to nature

1. Walk barefoot in nature

The root chakra, which is located at the end of your spine and which connects you into the Earth gives you a feeling of safety and protection when it's energetically strong. The quickest and easiest way to strengthen it is to simply take off your shoes and walk barefoot on the Earth.

The Earth's natural energy field is called "Schumann Resonance" and oscillates at 7.83 Hz. This is the energetic frequency your body thrives on and by making contact with it, your body and your energy centers will naturally go into a state of harmony and equilibrium.

2. Visualize the magical waterfall

If you cannot take a shower right away after interacting with stressful and energetically draining people or a situation, I suggest you practice the "magical waterfall" visualization. It's another one of my favorite ways to quickly cleanse my energy system.

Close your eyes and take a few deep breaths and simply imagine standing under a magical waterfall, which washes away any energies and impurities that don't belong to you. See and feel the warm water falling down onto your head, shoulders and running over your body until everything is washed away, leaving you energized and cleansed.

If you are new to visualization, it's important for you to know that you don't have to necessarily "see" everything clearly in your mind's eye for it to work. Just practice this visualization a few times and it will soon become second nature to you.

3. Visualize a Protective field around You

This is another simple, yet powerful exercise, which will strengthen your protective boundaries. However, before doing this visualization I strongly suggest you first cleanse your energy system as you don't want to "trap" energetic impurities in your system. Do this visualization when you are around lots of people, you are about to go into a particularly stressful situation or simply to increase your energetic and emotional resilience over time.

Take a few minutes and close your eyes. Now try to feel and sense your aura. Again, this might be hard to do in the beginning but with a little bit of practice it will become easier. Try to sense where your energetic boundaries end. Sometimes, your aura can be so open that it almost fills up the entire room. Sometimes it is much closer to the body.

What you want to do is to visualize and imagine your energetic boundaries stretching outward a few inches around your body. Once you can feel or sense it, visualize the energy around your body as dense and of a protective color. I have found that dark blue and purple are especially protective and work really well but you can play with it. Go with your instincts and intuition and use whatever color works best for you. You want to train yourself in such a way that you can **q**uickly and easily visualize the color around you so that you can quickly protect your energy field when you need it the most.

4. Take a sea salt shower or bath

One of my favorite ways to make sure my energy system is clear and cleansed is to simply take a shower with sea salt. Rub the salt into your skin while setting the intention to cleanse your aura, washing away anything that does not belong to you.

By using your intention, your consciousness directs the energy where it needs to go. You can also take a bath with sea salt. Simply add 4 cups of sea salt to the water and soak for 20 minutes. This simple method works like a charm and I guarantee you, you will feel better quickly. Since sea salt is such a good natural cleansing agent, I think this is the reason why so many people love swimming in the ocean. It's a natural aura cleanse.

One of my favorite ways to make sure my energy system is clear and cleansed is to simply take a shower with sea salt. Rub the salt into your skin while setting the intention to cleanse your aura, washing away anything that does not belong to you. By using your intention, your consciousness directs the energy where it needs to go.

You can also take a bath with sea salt. Simply add 4 cups of sea salt to the water and soak for 20 minutes. This simple method works like a charm and I guarantee you, you will feel better *q*uickly. Since sea salt is such a good natural cleansing agent, I think this is the reason why so many people love swimming in the ocean. It's a natural aura cleanse.

5. Strengthen your Root chakra

If you don't have the opportunity to walk barefoot in nature, the next best thing is to take your shoes off (you can do this inside your apartment), put your feet on the ground and visualize a grounding cord from the soles of your feet right into the Earth's center.
Do this for a few minutes until you feel more grounded and more at home within your body. Being grounding in your body is a natural protection against other people's energetic influence.

Chapter 12

KUNDALINI

Description

Everyone has an inner drive to excel or be special at something—to be unique. Sometimes people reach for this in negative ways. The underlying drive in all people, however, is one of evolution—to reach for enlightenment, to be God-like while still human. In the Upanishads, it is expressed: Dwelling in this very body, we have somehow realized Brahman [expansion, evolution, the Absolute, Creator, Preserver, and Destroyer of the universe]; otherwise we should have remained ignorant and great destruction would have overtaken us. Those who know Brahman become immortal while others only suffer misery. [IV, iv, 14/Swami Nikhilananda translation.] In the New Testament, Jesus answered: Is it not written in your own law, "I said: You are gods"? Those who are called gods to whom the word of God was delivered—and Scripture can not be set aside." [John 10:34-35/The New English Bible] We find that we are all called to go beyond our humanness toward greater heights. The Kundalini energy pushes each of us toward this goal of enlightenment—knowing the light, knowing God. In Tibetan Yoga and in other secret doctrines, it is expressed:

By means of Shakti Yoga [energy discipline], the Tantric yogin attains discipline of body and mind and then proceeds to the mighty task of awakening the dormant, or innate, powers of divinity within himself, personified as the sleeping Goddess Kundalini.... Then, from the mystic union of Shakta [at the top of the head] and the Shakti, is born Enlightenment; and the Yogin has attained the Goal.

Kundalini, a Sanskrit word meaning "circular power," is an individual's basic evolutionary force. Each of us is born with some of this energy already flowing. The amount available and usable determines whether a person has low intelligence, is a genius, or is somewhere in the middle. It is not just a matter of using what we already have, but of awakening the much greater amount waiting in the Kundalini reservoir located at the base of the spine. Kundalini is a natural force common to all of us. It is not a religion, although it is practiced by some religions and the process can enhance and develop each person's own religious beliefs.

Ancient Eastern literature contains a great deal of information on the Kundalini. This is not true of Western literature; but more is being written. As interest in the Aquarian Age grows rapidly and brings stronger energies to facilitate spontaneous Kundalini release, people in all walks of life, all ages and all levels of growth, experience Kundalini, regardless of cultural, philosophical or religious backgrounds. Little information is available for people who have not even heard of Kundalini and wonder at the causes of their physical, mental, or emotional suffering or breakdown. Even those in the growth and help fields do not have easy access to information for counseling those who release extra Kundalini before their systems are ready and experience problems on all levels of life, as if 220 energy suddenly coursed through their 110 units; fuses blow and circuitry melts. One reason for the lack of information is that many people, though knowledgeable, are concerned about the Kundalini power's potential for harm; they feel nothing should be done with it—no exercises and no training—because of the possibility that this awesome force will turn destructive. This attitude is much the same as that of people who say that if you don't educate children about sex, there won't be any problems. Another reason is that many people regard Kundalini as a new age fad. Nothing could be further from the truth. Kundalini can be considered the oldest known science.

In previous ages people raised Kundalini under the guidance of teachers and in controlled circumstances, preserving what they learned as an esoteric knowledge. But we have entered a period of time in which the esoteric becomes exoteric. People whose Kundalini was raised without their knowledge, relating symptoms of their condition to others, were generally considered crazy or physically weak; they may even have considered themselves crazy. The process may entail great confusion and fright beyond the exhilaration and sense of being uplifted. It is evident from their writings that Christian mystics had experiences of released Kundalini, which they referred to as sufferings. They understood the process as one which would bring union with God. Gopi Krishna has been a modem exponent of this evolutionary energy. His own Kundalini release came from meditation practices he undertook without prior formal training. He spent years working with and understanding what was happening to him. His experiences and writings have been very beneficial to others who have not had previous training.

Symptoms of early release

Since we are all individuals—with our own history, physical conditions, personal and spiritual development—Kundalini release acts differently with each of us. These are some of the symptoms which may indicate an excessive release of Kundalini, meaning before the system is ready:

- Unexplained illness;

- Erratic behavior;

- A feeling of "losing it" and difficulty coping with everyday life;

- Chills or hot flashes;

- Evidence of multiple personalities;

- Excessive mood swings: depression or ecstasy;

- Times of extreme dullness or brilliance;

- Loss or distortion of memory;

- Disorientation with oneself, others, work, or the world in general;

- Extremes in appearance (a person may fluctuate between looking years younger one moment and twenty years older a short time later);

Visual effects: seeing lights or colors, geometric shapes, scenes from past lives, or future events.

Purpose

Kundalini has its own sense of direction. Its natural flow is up the spine and out the top of the head; along that path it brings new awareness, new abilities, and transcendental states. Much as a plant reaches toward light, the Kundalini pushes us to reach for enlightenment; it removes any energy blocks in its way, thus causing symptoms such as those listed above. It will do its own thing. We can help or hinder the process.

A fully developed person will have exceptional paranormal gifts, great spiritual awareness and truly be considered genius or God-like. Each of us must deal with the Kundalini sooner or later; the more knowledgeable and ready we are, the more wonderful the experience will be.

How to release your Kundalini Energy

The release process: The Kundalini energy lies coiled at the base of the spine. Its release may be likened to waves, flames, pulsations or an uncoiling. The uncoiled portion seeks an outlet, normally through the spine up to the top of the head and out what is sometimes called the crown chakra. Chakra, a Sanskrit word meaning "wheel," refers to the various energy vortices on our etheric body. Sometimes the energy coils upward around the spine, again ending at the crown chakra. In the natural evolutionary process, a number of layers or waves are individually released during a lifetime, depending on a person's growth and readiness. The movement of the wave is so imperceptible most people are not aware of the activity, though they may be aware of some heat (energy movement) in the tailbone area prior to the release.

More sensitive people will feel the energy progress up the spine. They may feel pressure or pain as the energy encounters a blocked area; pain may also appear when the energy patterns are not normal. There are many layers of Kundalini waiting to be released. The action is similar to peeling off the outer edges of an onion. A person can release a few or many layers during a lifetime. People knowledgeable about the Kundalini force may choose to release more, thus speeding their evolution; in extreme cases, liquid fire or extreme heat may be released. The Kundalini, sometimes called shakti (divine spark of life force), begins its ascent from the base of the tailbone, where it is stored. As it rises up the spinal column and goes out the top of the head, it blends with the spiritual energy available in the universe. An energy combination then showers down over the body and travels throughout the system, aiding in refining and cleansing the cells. If the Kundalini is blocked in its upward flow by improper energy patterns or negativity, or by an improperly prepared or cleansed body, it may drop after several days and then begin a slow, painful ascent up the body again, cleaning and refining as it goes. This process can create much havoc and may cause physical, emotional or mental distress.

A person who releases a number of layers of energy at once may be in a beautiful state for days or even weeks- Such a person may have extra physical strength, beautiful new understandings, feelings of bliss or transcendental awareness, or a feeling of really having made it and achieving enlightenment He or she may even have a little spiritual pride. For most people, however, this state disappears and the Kundalini begins its cleansing process; then the person wonders why things are now so difficult and where the wonderful "stuff" went. The latter is the usual Pattern of Kundalini release; it is not a matter of the person "messing up" their growth. When energy blocks are severe enough, blissful states do not occur; the energy goes immediately into the cleansing.

Energy blocks are caused by locked-in attitudes or feelings or old emotional or mental scars. Poor posture and injuries can also create energy blocks. People who have prepared well by taking care of their bodies and raising spiritual awareness will accomplish Kundalini cleansing more quickly and easily; they realize benefits almost immediately and the Kundalini rising is a beautiful experience. But if the system is not ready for this powerful force, years may be required to complete the process.

Once released, there is NO TURNING BACK! It is impossible to reverse the process, though it can sometimes be slowed. If a person decides the growth is no longer desirable and tries to hold back this energy, congestion and illness may result, which may, in extreme cases, lead to death. One must learn to work with it, or in some cases just survive it, while the heavy cleansing takes place. The change is usually not a magical, total overnight operation; the energy may take as long as twenty or twenty-five years to complete cleansing and refinement sufficient for the psychic or spiritual gifts to unfold. When a person knows how to work with the energy, has a healthy body, mind and spirit and is ready, change occurs in a much shorter period of time. People in the midst of an active natural Kundalini flow, already using it, take less time to make the new Kundalini available for use. In each incarnation it is necessary to learn over again to control and use the energy. This is one of the main purposes of childhood; children need behavior and attitude guidance to use their energies appropriately. Permitting their energies to run uncontrolled causes problems in daily living and impedes further growth.

Cleansing the physical

One can use Kundalini on the physical level to achieve a healthier body. The technique of directing Kundalini having been learned, energy may be sent to different areas of the body for rejuvenation, healing and strengthening. Working with it, one develops a sense of how much to send to each area and how it works best. The exercise for Kundalini Movement and Chakra Cleansing on [page 55] is excellent for understanding how to guide the energy. Letting the Kundalini flow gently into the area needing healing—changing it to the quality of liquid silk—is very soothing; the frequency of the energy changes to one more conducive to general healing. Bathe a particular area in this energy. Next, diffuse the energy throughout the entire body. Several sessions a week will increase circulation, help release blocks and generally aid in maintaining a youthful body. Faced with a need for greater than normal physical exertion, fill your body with the power of Kundalini; breathe it throughout the entire body, let it flow through and then do the task. Practice with it to see how to handle and use it. When physically affected by the various aches and pains stemming from raised Kundalini effects, promote release with deep, peaceful breathing followed by massage in the affected area; allow thoughts and feelings to come to your consciousness. Such an open meditation can be most helpful. If you cannot, for some reason, massage the hurt area (perhaps it is too painful), focus your attention on that area instead; concentrate your energy there and go into the discomfort. Often the aches and pains will leave in a short while and you will develop a memory or awareness of what has occurred.

The Ultimate: The physical body, cleansed and refined by the Kundalini, will appear youthful and be very energetic. It will seldom be ill (or illness will be short), have great power, and be capable of paranormal feats.

Our feelings emanate from the emotional body. We feel anger there, frustration when our needs are not met. From the emotional body we learn to give and express love and caring, thus fulfilling our needs to be in relationships. The emotional body is very demanding; seeking fulfillment, if not directly, through various hidden ways. Feeling depleted or unable to express, it may seek gratification and balance in smoking, eating certain foods, irrational behavior or any number of other ways. When we keep direct contact with our emotions we can deal with these in better ways.

Cleansing the Emotional

As the Kundalini cleanses the emotional area, one may find that emotions are out of proportion to a given situation. There may be crying spells or other emotional states without apparent reason; the Kundalini is simply hitting a block full-force. One's usual reaction is to block again; it is much better to enter an open meditation, allowing thoughts and feelings to surface, thus letting the block release. The block may be related to the feeling level either of a past life or an earlier experience from this life. It may also represent a present problem. Sometimes it even relates to things which have not yet happened but have only begun to manifest through the system.

Emotional control

Emotions and feelings are just vibratory rates; changing the rates, we can change our emotions and feelings. As an exercise, feel your sadness as deeply as possible. Now turn the sadness to joy and try to notice a change of vibrational quality. Do the same with fear, turning it into faith and courage. Feel jealousy; turn that into understanding your own needs. Turn pride into thankfulness. Take any emotional *q*uality that is difficult for you, think of its opposite, and work with it in this manner. Learn to feel without getting caught in it. Keep a perspective on the situation by e*q*ualizing energies in the body. Feel energy in the back as well as the front; energy that remains primarily in the belly area creates a tendency in us to give far more attention to the feelings than they deserve. Massage the belly area and ask what is there that needs to be recognized; then move the energy into the entire body, to assimilate or eliminate it.

The Ultimate: After cleansing and refining, it is possible to have feelings without getting caught in them, to experience life without causing more karma and blocks, and to love without attachment. The emotional body will then give richness and depth to whatever you do.

The mental body contains matter which can vibrate at a rate similar to that of the creative force in our cosmos. It is where we begin to think, to reason, to know, to create. Through the mental body we gather knowledge; through reason and logic, we apply that knowledge. It is also through this body that we set up rigid attitudes or structures in our system. Here prejudices are formed. The more rigid the matter in our mental body becomes, the more difficult it is to flow with life, to learn new ways of living and to acquire new ideas.

Cleansing the mental

While the Kundalini cleanses the mental body, a person may find strong, previously unknown prejudices or become aware of life-governing attitudes which have long determined actions and reactions.

Clearing the Brain

Concentrate on breathing through your nose, up into your head. Look into your head as you would look up into the heavens and observe the stars in the sky. What colors, what energy patterns can you observe?

Truth

Do the Deep, Peaceful Breathing, concentrating on the center of your forehead; visualize the word "truth" in that area. Breathe in and feel truth enter your entire system, flooding each cell. Try to hold this in the system, while doing the Deep, Peaceful Breathing, for at least two minutes. During Kundalini cleansing it is especially easy for untruths and misconceptions (which block growth) to enter your thoughts. If you have mental work to do but your energy will not flow, try dancing. Dancing is excellent for releasing Kundalini flow and will aid in the thinking and intuitive processes. Since mental work is often done in a way that is not conducive to good Kundalini flow —at a desk or a table, curved over your work, shoulders rounded and hunched, head lowered—try to improve your posture and take breaks in which you walk, dance or exercise. Kundalini flow to the brain is slowed when you are caught in emotional situations and relationship problems (common, in this age). Having faith that "this too shall pass," and gaining perspective on the situation, helps keep energy flow open to the brain.

The Ultimate: You will think and create in new ways and work with higher dimensions. Manifestation and other mental powers will be considered normal.

Chapter 13

Aura

Aura

Science observes that galaxies are surrounded by massive halos of dark matter. Curiously a similar observation was made by a Hindu mystic, half a century ago. He too saw halos around galaxies - but they were anything but dark or invisible. He says:
"The divine dispersion of rays poured from an eternal Source, blazing into galaxies, transfigured with ineffable auras." - Paramahansa Yogananda, 1946
The term "aura" is frequently used in metaphysics to mean a colored radiation emanating from an object. Spherical halos around saints, as depicted in certain paintings, are considered auras around the head region. What were invisible halos to scientists appeared as a colorful aura around the galaxies to this saint, as he observed them half a century ago. Was he seeing what our scientific instruments could not see - the dark matter counterparts of these galaxies? Paramahansa Yogananda also observed in 1946 that the "astral luminaries resemble the aurora borealis". Based on plasma metaphysics, it is easy to see that the aura is generated in a similar process as the aurora.

The Aurora

Kristian Birkeland put forward the auroral theory which is now widely accepted by scientists. According to him, electrically charged particles ejected from sunspots are captured by Earth's magnetic field and directed along the field's lines into the polar regions. The charged particles follow spiral or helical tracks about the lines of force. The incoming particles excite the atoms and molecules in the air and ionize them - stripping them into their non-neutral constituents. This results in the colorful displays that are associated with auroras.

Birkeland used a simple device to prove his theory - he placed a sphere containing an electromagnet inside a large vacuum chamber, which represented the space around the Earth and its magnetic field. He then shot clouds of electrons toward this simulated Earth to produce a light phenomenon that looked like the aurora. This configuration is exactly the same as in a subtle body, as explained below.

Anatomy of the Subtle Body

According to plasma metaphysics, the subtle body is a body of magnetic plasma (or "magma"). It sits inside an ovoid which has a plasma "auric" sheath around it (equivalent to the sphere in the Birkeland device) and contains a magnetized central channel (equivalent to the electromagnet in the Birkeland device).

How is the Aura generated?

The aura that is radiated by a subtle body is generated by a procedure not unlike the one that generates the aurora borealis. There is a tendency for charged particles to follow magnetic lines of force. The energetic charged super particles (identified as "qi", "prana" or "kundalini" particles) rush towards the various nodes of the chakras (which contain intense magnetic fields) at very high speeds. They spiral around helical paths just before they are absorbed by the chakras near the head and feet (the "poles") and other chakras around the body. While doing so, they generate a light phenomenon in the subtle bodies - very much like that of the aurora borealis.

Anyone who compares the Kirlian images (or representations) of human auras (or who can actually see them) with the aurora borealis will no doubt find a strong resemblance. However, while the aurora is a natural plasma light show comprising standard particles (i.e. particles described in the physicists' "Standard Model") - the aura is a natural plasma light show of super (i.e. supersymmetric) particles!

The electromagnetic processes that give rise to the aurora borealis are the same as those which give rise to the human aura. If this is accepted, then it also confirms that subtle bodies are composed of a magnetic plasma of super particles - which is currently classified under dark matter.

Protecting and Cleansing your Aura

Your aura is like your energetic protective force field that not only protects you, but it also allows you to shine your light outward. Have you ever felt someone's presence before even knowing they enter a room or say anything? It is probably because you felt their aura and what it is giving off.

Of course you want people to feel your True essence if you are someone who is not afraid for others to see who you truly are.

Your aura acts like an energetic magnet as well. When it is not cleansed, it can collect debris to the point that it gets weakened and not as proficient.

When your aura gets weakened, your body is susceptible to unwanted energy that can lead to sickness.

Energy Healers

Sometimes your aura can be broken down from pollution and smoke-filled environments, chemicals, computers, Internet, negative thinking and partaking in negative-like behavior or activities that lower your frequency.

Besides the pollution and environmental aspects, the negative thought patterns can actually be from years of built up unwanted energy that has unbalanced us emotionally and in all other aspects as well. A great and effective way to change these patterns is to ask for Divine guidance to assist us in letting go of all energetic baggage. This will help us break old patterns and cycles of behavior that do not serve us anymore.

Sea salt bath

Salt and water are both great and natural purifying and cleansing agents for energetic debris.

Fill a bathtub with warm water and place a couple hand-fulls of salt (sea salt, bath salts, etc) in the water to dissolve.

Lay in the bathtub with the intent of all energetic debris being released and your aura strengthening and being cleansed.

As this process is happening, why not make it a meditative moment with soft music and candles. Just relax!

Cold water showers

Cold water is another natural way to cleanse our energetic field (chakras and aura). Not only does it cleanse the energy body, but it also does the following:

- uplifts the mood
- boosts energy levels
- speeds up the healing process
- improves circulation
- detoxes your body (removes toxins)
- helps to clear negative thinking

Cold showers may feel uncomfortable at first, but you can actually build a tolerance to this. Make sure to only do these a few seconds at a time at first and then build up to minutes at a time. Try not to shock your system.

CONCLUSION

Chakras and other body energies regulate your body energy levels, and how energy moves throughout. Chakras influence our decisions we make. Although Chakras are not a "physical" element of the body, they do have many physical influences. They interact with the body through the glandular or Endocrine System. Chakras are assigned to seven Endocrine Glands as well as with groupings of nerve bundles called nerve plexuses.

The Chakras correspond with states of consciousness, personality types and endocrine secretions. Science is now confirming that different colors interact with the endocrine system of the body to stimulate or inhibit hormonal production. Hormones directly affect our physical, emotional, and mental states. In fact, color travels through the eyes directly to the brain's hypothalamus and through the Supra Chiasmatic Nucleus to affect over 400 various functions within the body.

Color therapy is often used to treat the Chakra system through various treatment methods. By knowing your personal colors and your own Chakra system, you will be able to enhance your health, your life reactions and decisions, and your overall quality of life.

To be able to harness the properties of color, light is the natural tool of choice for color therapy. Energy Healing has been around for Millennia. The shamans and healers and priests of countless world cultures already know the power of vibration. However, modern man is just catching up. The scientific study of Energy Healing is in it's infancy and it's surprising how little research has been done. What we have done is compile as much of the existing research as we could into this section, and added in our own studies.

Despite the truly astounding discoveries that have been made about the science of energy healing, the traditional scientific and medical communities still seem to regard energy work as a theoretical and fanciful concept. It's time for that to change!

As Seven Chakras are 7 specific energy center points in our energetic fields.   When the chakras are balanced energy flows into and out of each of these 7 centers harmoniously. When they are out of balance the energy can become blocked in one or more of the chakra points. This causes the energetic patterns of the body to flow too quickly or too slowly. The concept of chakras comes from India and is thousands of years old. Extensive references to the chakra system are in the Upanishads, the Hindu holy books written in 1000 BC. Modern medicine has yet to validate the subtle energetic centers of the chakra system, but we're hoping they catch up soon. In the meantime, those who have balanced their chakras know how powerful these energy centers are.

Note from the author :

Thank you for reading this book. We have also created a - Guided Meditation for Chakra Awakening by Healeanor Crystal, that you can find on Audible. If you are a beginner, I suggest you follow that one combined with all the knowledge in this book, for faster results.